Jane Wenham-Jones is a well-
who regularly appears on radio
a wide variety of magazines and newspapers, including
My Weekly, *Woman's Weekly* and as the agony aunt for
Writing Magazine.

She has published six novels: *Raising The Roof*, *Perfect
Alibis*, *One Glass Is Never Enough*, *Prime Time*, *Mum in
the Middle* and *The Big Five O*, as well as two previous
how-to books: *Wannabe a Writer?* and *Wannabe a Writer
We've Heard Of?*

Jane lives with her family in Broadstairs, Kent, where three
of her novels are set.

For more info see www.janewenham-jones.com and
www.wannabeawriter.com

Also by Jane Wenham-Jones and available from Headline

Non-fiction:
Wannabe a Writer?
Wannabe a Writer We've Heard Of?

Fiction:
Raising the Roof
Perfect Alibis
One Glass Is Never Enough
Prime Time
Cat Tales for Cat Lovers
Something to Celebrate
Happy Birthday

100 Ways To Fight The Flab

And Still Have Wine and Chocolate

JANE WENHAM-JONES

ACCENT

First published in 2013 by ACCENT PRESS LTD

This edition published in 2020 by Headline Accent,
an imprint of HEADLINE PUBLISHING GROUP

1

Illustrations by Jane Wenham-Jones
Except for "Buy a doreen" (p.177) "Wear a tent" (p.178) and
"Boxing with weights" (p.159) by Shirley Webb
Back cover photograph by Bill Harris

Cataloguing in Publication Data is available from the British Library

ISBN 978 1 4722 8031 2

Offset in 11/15 pt Times New Roman by Jouve (UK), Milton Keynes

Printed and bound in Great Britain by Clays Ltd, Elcograf S.p.A.

HEADLINE PUBLISHING GROUP
An Hachette UK Company
Carmelite House
50 Victoria Embankment
London
EC4Y 0DZ

www.headline.co.uk
www.hachette.co.uk

CONTENTS

INTRODUCTION

This book started out as a bit of a joke.

It began life as a spin-off from the chapter in my how-to book *Wannabe a Writer?* that advised on Writer's Bottom – a term I take full credit for coining – which is an occupational hazard associated with spending long hours welded to the computer while failing to take enough exercise or eat anything other than chocolate. (Some authors complain of Writer's Stomach, Chins, and Upper Arms too.)

Written mostly to amuse myself, and perhaps give fellow scribes a smile, this small e-publication, available on Kindle, was advertised as containing one hundred "hilarious" suggestions for keeping a spreading rear at bay.

The tips were all intended to be light-hearted, but almost as soon as I'd finished recording them, I realised how seriously I take them.

Number one was "Eat Chocolate". That's got to be a joke, right? Actually, no. I eat chocolate every day. It is one of my chief weight-control tactics (as well as being a fine excuse). I rather like crisps too.

I wrote then that I am probably not thin enough to be writing a diet book – if thin means having no bum and legs like twigs. But nor am I obese. Weight charts rate me as "normal"; I have a BMI of under 22, a hip-to-waist ratio that passes muster with the medical profession and I have, when wearing black and the sort of underwear that crushes your internal organs, even been described as "slim".

Which, considering my unhealthy career choice, vast consumption of wine and nibbles, and somewhat erratic approach to exercise, is, you might say, a small miracle.

Except it isn't. It is the simple result of a set of strategies I have learned to rely on to keep tubbiness at arm's length. So that if I want to, I can eat junk food and still fit into a tight dress.

This is not a diet book.

I am not thin enough to write a diet book so this isn't one. I bet that's not the first time you've heard that!

The authors may call it an "Eating Plan", a "Whole New Approach", or put the emphasis on a change of "Lifestyle". But scratch the surface of most get-thin books and underneath they've all got the same bad news. You've got to stop eating anything nice!

Typically, there's a skinny bird on the front cover, or some mumbo-science on the back and a strap line telling you you'll never go hungry. They use words like "permanent" and "healthy". They tell you that after reading these particular pearls of wisdom, you *need never go on a diet again* ...

At this point, you know that's going to be bunkum. You might not be going on their definition of "diet" but do any of these fine works, on any of their 350 pages (largely

2

comprised of repeating themselves and giving endless recipes for steamed dullard with low-fat, sugar-free, tedium dressing), ever recommend sitting down with a bottle of Chablis and a packet of Kettle Chips? Do they suggest on Day Four of *Lose a Stone and Never Feel Hungry* that a Danish pastry is the way to go? Any mention of it being just fine to mop up fourteen cold chips and half a fish finger from the kids' plates?

I think not.

Whichever way you look at it, it is all about cutting out.

Books like that occasionally allow a "Daily Treat". One fun-sized Mars Bar, say, or a small glass of dry white wine.

What's fun about a chocolate bar an inch long? Where is the joy in knowing before you start you are restricted to *one* glass of wine?

We're not stupid. However much we may bluster about slow metabolisms and big bones and layers of lard running in the family, even those of us with absolutely zilch in the understanding-science department, can secretly grasp the basic equation regarding portions in and expenditure of energy out. Namely:

If what goes in is greater than what goes out, you get fat.

If what goes in equals what goes out, you stay the same (this may equal above).

If what goes in is less than the sum of what goes out you get thin (hurrah!).

Though maybe not "hurrah" for long, because, as entire volumes on the perils of yo-yo dieting have hastened to tell us, the moment you go back to eating anything at all that you like, you'll be waddling again.

3

Depressing, innit?

That's why there's all this emphasis on a "change of lifestyle". It's short-hand for never, ever, eat what you really want again.

I am here to tell you, you can. I am here to tell you there is, dear reader, *another way* ...

And I will share it with you.

But first, as a disclaimer, I must point out that I am not a nutritionist, or a doctor, and if you are truly massive and needing three airline seats there is little I can do except to suggest you don't wear white leggings. (And hope that there is perhaps one tip in this book that speaks to you and helps you turn things around – especially with the cost of air travel these days!)

Also, in fairness, I should tell you, I have never been HUGE.

I can't offer you stories about how I topped twenty-five stone and had to be winched out of the hotel bath after I'd broken the bed.

Instead, I have spent a lot of my life at the sort of weight where, if I've dressed cleverly, held my stomach in and made sure I'm not snapped with a wide-angled lens, I've managed to get by without anybody thinking I'm too much of a fat moo (heavy weekend on the peanuts, a badly cut dress, and the skinniest friend in tow: different story).

But I always weighed just that bit more than I wanted to be. I have seen photos of myself that have made me shudder (Google-image me – you'll see what I mean), and there have been phases of my life when I've carried very definite layers of podge – where even if I've got it well covered,

4

I've known about the flabby bits round my middle and have longed for just the one chin and spaghetti arms.

I've felt miserable on the mornings when I've weighed more, guilty when I knew it was all my own fault for being weak-willed, pleased with myself when I've lost a bit and when it's been really, really important to me, I have put my mind to losing half a stone. Which I then, invariably, put back on the moment I went back to "normal".

Why? Because there are two big reasons why all diets/eating plans/changes of lifestyle eventually fail. And that is, that unless you have a will of iron and a very high tolerance to emotional and physical discomfort (in which case you are probably already as thin as a rake and won't be reading this book anyway) they all involve feeling either hungry or deprived or both. It is no wonder that nobody sticks to a diet for long and the overweight have a whole shelf load of books promising dramatic weight loss, have tried them all, and are still waddling round the house with a KitKat in each hand.

Because it is pretty dispiriting for anyone to face a future in which there is a stark choice between waving goodbye to the notion of cake for the next twenty years or getting your jeans up past your knees.

If you can get round those twin problems of hunger and feeling that you're missing out, you can be the weight you want for ever. And you'll find it much easier to cope with either one of them, if you do have to, if you know that feeling will be short-lived. Weight loss is a question of attitude as much as what you put in your mouth – a case, if you like, of mind over large quantities of matter.

In this book, I will share my tips on shifting the flab in the first place, if that's what you need to do, but, more importantly, on keeping to a happy weight afterwards, while still actually having *a life*.

(For me, that means being able to have a drink, eat chocolate, and go out to dinner with friends without being a tedious pain in the *derrière*.) Because there is a middle way between living on tissue paper and being as thin as a stick, and eating what makes you happy and watching the pounds pile on.

I am still not as totally sylph-like as I might dream of being – because one is never satisfied – but my weight doesn't fluctuate by more than a couple of pounds and I get into all my clothes – even the garments I've had for over a decade. If I've got an event coming up and am feeling extra vain, if there will be a lot of photos taken and/or the frock I'll be wearing is particularly unforgiving, I can shed a few pounds quite quickly – see the section entitled **Shift it Fast** – but for the rest of the time I eat, drink, make merry, and still manage to fit my Writer's Bottom into just the one chair.

Here's how.

GETTING STARTED ON FLAB-FIGHTING

By this, I don't mean you have to do anything right now. You can go and get a chocolate biscuit if you want and settle yourself comfortably and indulge in a little reverie about what you are going to eat for dinner. Yes, chips are fine (maybe have a side salad too – vitamins are always good) – there is no need to start to fret about what you have to give up because you don't have to say goodbye to anything. Not for ever, anyway.

Keep that in mind, because the thought of giving up anything permanently is likely to evoke immediate feelings of misery and loss.

I can remember thinking, when I was a smoker, that if I should never put another cigarette in my mouth, my life wouldn't be worth living. (That was over twenty years ago and of course I am entirely delighted to be a non-smoker now.)

If you have a serious alcohol dependency, then the advice is going to be to turn your back on the booze for ever. And many diet books seem to take the similar view that if you're an overweight over-eater you should train yourself to treat chocolate cake like a dangerous drug. I don't agree.

There is no doubt that a sugar overload is bad for you for all sorts of reasons, but you don't want to start your new way of approaching what you eat by feeling miserable.

If you usually begin a diet and immediately start thinking of all the stuff you're going to miss out on, you can relax because this time you're not. Because a) we're going to be realistic about what we can do and when we can do it, and b) because we are going to deal with any sense of deprivation we feel.

Instead of feeling fed up already, you should be feeling happy and thrilled and hugely grateful (no worries, you can thank me later) because you're going to have a great time, keep your weight down without worrying, and eat chocolate without guilt. Hurrah!

You are going to be slimmer.

Or the "slimmer" that works for you. Because Rule No 1 is: be realistic. About yourself and what is achievable. For while it is desirable to be fit and healthy, there is no point feeling despondent and guilty about one's natural shape. Especially, if you are female and using women from the fashion pages as your role model.

Any diet that attempts to give us a figure that only about three per cent of women are actually genetically programmed to have is going to take up far too much concentration and energy, be exceedingly dispiriting and dull, and you would basically have to stay on it for ever. Look at the malnourished twig-people, wafting up the catwalk wearing clothes that you or I couldn't get one leg in – do they look happy?

Being realistic is the key.

You may have no desire to look like a stick, anyway, but simply want to be a little fitter and less flabby round the edges. I have no wish to be the Fat Police (nor am I in a position to be!). Big does not preclude beautiful and I am quite comfortable with the argument that being overweight is only a problem if it is making you unhappy or affects your health.

After all, *very* thin people may look lovely in magazines but in real life they can be quite annoying. You wonder why they bother going to a restaurant at all just to suck on a piece of lettuce; and who wants a non-wheat, non-dairy, can't-eat-fat, what's-its carb-content, I hope-there's-no-sugar-in-that, teetotaller round to dinner? Nice, fun, rounded guests are much more the ticket.

In fact, a few years back, I conceived a book called **Bugger the Diet and Everything Else Life's Too Short For.**

When this was, sadly, not fallen upon by an eager publishing world I contented myself with putting an extract up on my website, together with the following illustrated chart, entitled "How Fat Are You?" – the sub-text being: And does it really matter? It looked like this:

How Fat ARE you? Do you look like:

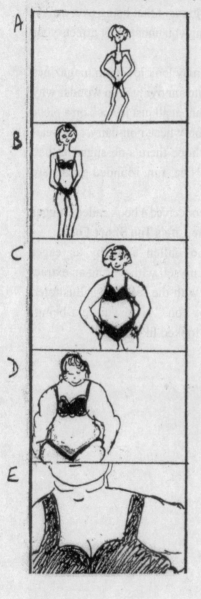

A) An anorexic stick insect. What are you doing reading a book with Diet in the title? Go get help.

B) Only 4% of women look like this and boy do they suffer for it. No chocolate, no wine, no crisps, no deep crust pizza with extra toppings. Do you want to be a miserable cow?

C) Not perfect but average. And what's wrong with that?

D) Soft and voluptuous. Men love it!

E) Yeah, OK, getting a bit obese here but nothing a floor-length tent wouldn't put right

Ha, ha hilarious etc. I went on to remind my readers that whoever first said that older women had to choose between their figures or their faces was spot on. A bit of fat does make you look younger.

And even if you are young already, I reasoned, you might as well be prepared.

I have since discovered that having a big bottom, for example, can actually be a healthy life choice – research carried out at Oxford University found that those with plenty of gluteofemoral fat – that's a lard arse to you and me – have a lower risk of diabetes, while further studies have shown that the owners of a fat bum are set for a riper old age than those with a ballooning belly.

(Not so great for those **with** the large belly but it does go to show that not all excess weight is a terrible thing). Indeed when you are very old – so old, I suspect that your face has had it, whatever the scales say – it is generally agreed that it is better longevity-wise to be a little over-weight than under.

And, at any age, just because you're not size zero and have never been mistaken for Kate Moss, it doesn't mean you're an elephant with a weight issue.

I wasted a lot of time in my youth thinking all the problems in my life would dissolve away if only I lost a stone. (It takes a few years to learn that in reality what really improves things is to ditch the dodgy boyfriend, get a job you actually like, and do anything at all to boost your self-esteem – more of that later.)

But there is also no doubt that being slimmer feels very nice and that we all want to lose the flab and shape up from time to time – after Christmas and Easter; before the summer; when a wedding's coming up or your thin friend is having a party; any time one needs to bare arms.

Presumably if you've bothered to open this book, you do too. And think how good it would be if you could then stay like that without getting bored and disgruntled.

So my outlook has altered a little. But since art is not my strong point, and I still have a lot of book to write, it seems a shame to waste the drawings. So I am using the same ones again on which I have updated my thoughts. Which are that, actually, sometimes, being overweight does matter – particularly, as we've said, if it upsets you or is adversely affecting your health.

I'm all for being large and bonny if those on the hefty side are happy with that. But considering this is just one of about a zillion books on the market right now on the subject of how to shift the lard, and the diet industry as a whole is worth billions of pounds, I can only assume not many are.

So let's look at this new chart instead:

How Fat ARE you? Do you look like:

A		Nothing's changed for me here. Women (and men!) **can** be too thin. You shouldn't be looking at a book with flab in the title either. Go eat a bun!
B		Of course you want to look like this. So do I – who wouldn't? It can be done but will take discipline, commitment and a lot of hunger-management and overcoming your sense of deprivation (see sections on same). How much do you want it?
C		Can you settle for this? This is easy. And once you've read up on the above and got your head round it you could end up closer to B than C anyway. Esp with your clothes <u>on</u>. (See section on hold-it-all-in garments.)
D		It's true that men like women with "a bit of padding" but do you? Are you comfortable? Happy with the way your trousers fit? If not, stick with me kid, we can do it... ☺
E		A floor-length tent will indeed cover a multitude of sins but it's really not good for you being that big, is it? This book is going to change your life. So start razzing yourself up and getting excited NOW ☺ ☺

13

Yes, I mean it. *Get excited*!

Because you are going to lose weight reading this book and then you are going to keep that weight off for a long, long time. (I won't say for ever because that's what they all say and by the time you're ninety, you might decide that a peaceful death by chocolate cake is what you want.)

But for now – you are going to be slim. Let us sum up and focus for a moment on why:

Ten great things about being slimmer.

1 You feel better. When you lose weight, there is quite literally a lightness about you. You will find you move more quickly, with a spring in your step. You will feel more confident so you will stand up straighter and smile more and when you do both these things you will look even better.

2 You can wear a much greater range of clothing without going into meltdown when you look in the mirror.

3 You can drift around with a doughnut hanging out of your mouth, pretending to be one of those infuriating, naturally skinny people with a metabolism on overdrive who eat all day long and never put on an ounce. (NB if you dig beneath the surface of the lifestyles of same, you will find that they in fact do a lot of things outlined in this book – sometimes without even realising.)

4 You can run, jump, hop, skip, without puffing like a steam engine. This in turn will make you even slimmer.

5 Your son will stop talking to you in the voice of Matt Lucas's Marjorie from *Little Britain*'s Fat-fighters, and shrieking *cake* and "Get that in your fat gob …" every time you open the biscuit tin. (NB this might just be in my house.)

6 You will be healthier, and lower your risk of getting all sorts of nasties in later life. (NB if you are already in later life, it is not too late to make it easier on your body from now on.)

7 You'll only need one airline, theatre, or cinema seat and the metal safety bar things on the rides will fit over your stomach should you go to a theme park. Small children will not point and laugh if you wedge yourself into the roller-coaster chair but fail to get out. Nor will the fire brigade be called. (And if they are, the nice fireman who rescues you will be able to throw you over his shoulder – mmm ☺)

8 There'll be no more gross pictures of you popping up on Facebook when you least expect it (don't you just love those sort of "friends" with cameras?)

9 There'll be room for you in that crowded lift or on the tube in the rush-hour.

10 If do you go mad and eat a whole chocolate gateau, three-tier pizza, and a bucket of pork-scratchings with a battered Mars Bar, at least you'll have a bit of leeway there and won't actually explode.

You might have your own reason for wanting to be thinner and be able to think up extra benefits I haven't listed.

E.g. the next time you bump into your ex, you will be able to sashay/swagger past looking amazing, sculpted, toned, and entirely yummy and irresistible and leaving him/her pig sick about letting you go when you are so much more alluring than the new partner (who will also be there looking rather tired and flabby).

OR: Your husband/wife will have to stop calling you Podge because you have now clearly have a waist the circumference of his/her thigh.

OR you will be able to finally fit into that hugely expensive but rather optimistically purchased dress/suit you bought five years ago in a size too small, because it was reduced.

OR you can now pinch your sister's clothes and get her back for the way she always takes your shoes.

Write your own most pressing reason for wanting to become and stay slim here:

And hold that thought!

Are you holding it? Yes, I hear you cry, but I've done all this before. Of course you have. A good friend made me laugh when she told me that the "fat" photo of herself she'd once pinned to her fridge door as a reminder to lose weight, was now there to illustrate her target! (A lesson on counting one's blessings at the time – I wouldn't mind being the weight I was when I was twenty-five and thought I was gross or to look as I did when I was thirty and fretting about all my "wrinkles".) However much we might long to be thinner, have the incentives and know all the theory, in practice we start our diets with high hopes and we still give up and give in and buy the next size up. Why?

KNOW YOUR ENEMIES: HUNGER, DEPRIVATION, AND BOREDOM

I said there were two reasons why diets fail – I should perhaps have made it three.

If you are hungry, or feeling a sense of deprivation, or are just plain bored, you won't stick to any sort of eating plan for more than a few days – or even hours.

Wanting to put food in our mouths is a primal instinct and the feeling of actual hunger – as opposed to the feeling of "mmm – that smells good, I could just do with a burger and large fries, even though I had lunch an hour ago" – is hard to ignore.

There are ways to manage it, suppress it, and turn it to your advantage which we will look at later, but as we know it is basically a protective mechanism to prevent you from starving to death (unlikely as that scenario is in the obesity-ridden Western world) and your body's way of telling you, via contraction of the stomach muscles and the release of gastrointestinal hormones, that it needs sustenance.

All your natural impulses are geared up to giving that body what it wants, so you shouldn't feel too guilty if you can't resist them. And you shouldn't ignore them for too long either. If you are feeling wobbly or dizzy, can't concentrate, have a headache or stomach cramps, then for heaven's sake eat something. Go and do it now!

There is however, a big difference between real hunger and just fancying something because you are bored or tired, or it looks nice, or you've had one and now you've got the taste in your mouth you find you can easily consume six.

It is a little like the old adage about the difference between having a cold and flu. Men, of course, always suffer from the latter, but for women, it boils down to what you would do if someone left a grand on your front lawn. If you'd get out of bed and retrieve it, you've got a cold. If you still couldn't manage to make it down the stairs, it's probably flu.

If you were really starving, you'd tuck in gratefully to all the things you'd usually approach with caution – say liver (ugh) or banana custard (yuck) – fill in your own *bêtes noires* as applicable – and if truly at death's door, munch on your grandmother.

But if the only thing you fancy is a packet of crisps or a jam doughnut then you are probably simply peckish or a bit sugar-depleted.

That is not to say you can't have said snack – if you can balance it out later – but it is worth holding on to the difference between the two feelings.

I believe a lot of people are overweight because they've actually lost their ability to discern proper hunger, and now ignore, or don't even notice, the signals of satiety.

In order to keep your weight down you either need to avoid hunger or harness it as a power for good and turn it to your advantage. (More of that in the later section – imaginatively entitled: **How to deal with hunger.)**

But it's not always feeling hungry that's the problem.

Let us say you are on a low-fat diet, involving lots of

plain baked potatoes and pasta without a creamy sauce, dry wholemeal toast and salad (no dressing), etc. You probably won't be hungry because those foods are filling and have a low rating on the GI index, meaning they release their energy slowly, but very soon you may well feel deprived.

Because, however much the diet sheet entreats you to add flavour with pepper or herbs, fat-free dressing (always unpleasant) or spices, baked potatoes are only really nice with butter and grated cheese; plain pasta is dull, and toast without butter is, frankly, a travesty. So the moment you see someone else tucking into a buttery crumpet, dolloping the mayonnaise onto their chips or having a spaghetti carbonara, you are going to start feeling sorry for yourself and deprived. Even if you hold out, sooner or later the temptation will become too much, and you'll think "sod it" and pour cream on your apple crumble.

If your regime allows fat but cuts out the carbohydrates and sugars, you may well enjoy your steak with hollandaise sauce, your egg and bacon and don't-hold-the-sausage breakfasts, and start out thoroughly enthusiastic about your nightly cheese platter. But, sooner or later, you will find yourself unable to think about anything except how much you'd like a sandwich and if you're invited out for tea to where there are homemade biscuits and a particularly luscious-looking cake, you may feel equally hard done by if you have to sit there with only a lump of cheddar.

If you're simply cutting calories and have committed yourself to a routine of living on yoghurt and fruit and chicken salad and crispbreads, washed down with water, how are you going to feel when you go out to dinner with the friends who believe in three courses, 1000-cal puddings, and chocolate mints with the port once the wine bottles are all empty?

And nobody (except the naturally teetotal) should be expected to go to a wedding or a big birthday and say no to champagne.

Sooner or later, hunger or deprivation (or plain fed-up-ness) will knock us off the dietary wagon and have us stuffing our faces with abandon.

So how do we avoid these twin evils, enjoy ourselves, and yet not end up the size of a house?

I'll tell you. We do not pin our colours to any one diet plan or even have a plan at all. We have a collection of strategies and tactics – think of it as a big bright bucket we can dip into – that we adapt to our individual lives and what works for US.

The problem with how-to books on so many subjects (and I speak as one who writes them) – from how to write a novel, to how to bring up children, to how to lose weight – is that they are generally so damn bossy.

Plot the whole of your story out first, they command, using colour-coded index cards and a spread-sheet. Ban sugar, limit TV, and put them on the naughty step. Raise your heartbeat for twenty minutes, three times a week and never eat cheese at the same meal as red meat. And so on.

Many diets consist of a series of instructions: you must eat this, must cut out that, and under no circumstances be tempted by a second helping of the other. But, when losing weight, as with so many things in life, there is no one size fits all (literally!) and the only route to lasting success in anything is to find our own way.

Mine is to tailor the way I eat, what exercise I do, and how much chocolate I get down my neck according to what's going on in my life that week and what appeals to me.

I have a short attention span, am easily bored and my levels of self-discipline cannot always be relied on. So I don't want to feel pinned down to the same eating and exercise patterns week in and week out. You may be different.

WHAT WILL WORK
FOR YOU?

You also need to be realistic about what you can manage.

We are all individual and therefore we are going to suit different sorts of diets. Some people can easily give up sugar but feel bereft if they're not allowed bread. Others need breakfast the moment they open one eye while others can happily last till lunch time on half an apple.

A friend of mine finds it really easy to survive on fruit all day long. If she wants to lose a few pounds or fit into a certain dress she just chomps on oranges and plums, strawberries and bananas from dawn to dusk. I cannot do this.

I once tried the grape diet (that's it – you just eat grapes – munching pips an' all if they have pips) and was going out of my head with the tedium of it by about 11 a.m.

David Headley, literary agent and owner of the fab Goldsboro Books, told me that he'd heard one can live perfectly well on champagne and carrots and still get all the nutrients you need.

I found this hard to believe and tried researching it on Google. I have ended up none the wiser but did discover a recipe for carrots cooked with dill that claimed it was useful for using up "left-over champagne" – who in their right minds has that??

I do know, however, that even if the carrots and fizz thing were true, it wouldn't do it for me. If I tried to live on bubbly I would pretty soon be needing crisps or a sandwich.

But I digress. As I was saying, a diet where I had endless fruit, and that was it, would just make me bad-tempered. On the other hand, I can go all day on cheese, nuts, and other little protein snacks with the odd cherry tomato thrown in, easily. In fact, once I get into the groove of a high-protein, low-carb regime, I feel positively great on it and develop the same sort of inner glow that others get from surviving on blueberry smoothies.

Stop here and make a list of the foods you really feel you cannot do without, those you can take or leave, those you could easily give up indefinitely, etc.

Fill this chart in now before you turn the page. (Oh dear, I'm getting bossy now too.)

I can't do without:	I can take or leave:	I can easily do without/ don't eat anyway	I'll be seriously bad-tempered if I don't get a daily fix of:	I should include:

If your chart looks like this:

I can't do without:	I can take or leave:	I can easily do without/ don't eat anyway	I'll be seriously bad-tempered if I don't get a daily fix of:	I should include:
Meat	Fruit	Breakfast cereal	Gin and tonic with peanuts	More vegetables
fish	sweets	Fizzy drinks		
Strange animal parts in general	Cakes chips			
Nuts				
Cheese				

Then obviously a high protein, low carb diet was heaven sent for you (and quite frankly I can't understand why you need to fight the flab in the first place, unless you are eating an entire cow with a whole bottle of Gordon's and your own bodyweight in roasted nuts.)

On the other hand if your chart looks more like this next one:

I can't do without:	I can take or leave:	I can easily do without/ don't eat anyway	I'll be seriously bad-tempered if I don't get a daily fix of:	I should include:
Bread crisps	Potatoes	Meat Fish poultry	Chocolate	Cheese, lentils and nuts as am vegetarian
	Pasta	Walnuts		
	Butter	Cabbage		
	Cake	Parsnips		
	Biscuits	Milk & cream		
	Fruit			

Then clearly the prospect of a regime that's all about cutting out sugar and carbs and eating lots of steak in a cream sauce and having no fruit isn't going to fill you with unalloyed joy. Worth bearing in mind when deciding on what tips will work for you.

27

On the other hand, sometimes putting up with a small amount of discomfort can pay huge dividends, and while it sounds all very anal and boring, keeping a proper food diary, with which to analyse the sort of eater you are, can be useful. This is because:

1   You can feel thoroughly disgusted with yourself when you see in black and white that you ate three pork pies before breakfast.
2   If you include a column for how you felt – energised, tired, bloated, grumpy, etc. it might help you track down your "food intolerances" – Ah ha! It is when I eat celery hearts after pigs' trotters that I go particularly blotchy – or:
3   You can study it carefully so as to do something very effective indeed in the battle of the bulge: Define your Downfall (see Tip No. 56).

So even if you only do it for one day (though a week would be better and give a clearer picture of your eating patterns) do try keeping a record of everything you consume and why.

NB this is most useful of all if you keep a diary of what you eat when left to your own devices – i.e. you are not attempting to lose weight but just following your natural instincts. So if you want to delay starting to fight your flab for a tad longer, and have another sausage roll, now's your chance ☺. If you want to get on with getting slim right away, perhaps you can remember what you ate yesterday (if so you're a better man/woman than I am!) But however you do it, I'd like you to make a chart a bit like this:

Day of Week : *Thursday*

Time	Where I was	What I ate	What I drank	Any mitigating circumstances
7.30am	Home	2 slices of toast and marmite	Tea	
11am	work	Jam doughnut	coffee	Bertha's birthday
1pm	Café near work	Egg and cress sandwich & crisps	Mineral water	
3pm	work	Slice cake	coffee	Still Bertha's birthday – she'd have been hurt if I'd refused
4-6pm			water	
6.30pm	Bar round corner	Bag peanuts	Cocktails then wine	Bertha – you know what she's like if you don't celebrate with her
8.30pm	still there		more	See above
9pm	Kebab shop by bus stop	Bag chips	water	About to fall over if not eat something
10pm	Home	Cheese, biscuits, crisps, half a tomato, bit of last night's cold pasta, half tub houmous on crispbread, another tomato, 2 chocolate biscuits	Water, black coffee, small red wine, more coffee and another glass of water	
2am			Water	

Day of Week : *Friday*

Time	Where I was	What I ate	What I drank	Any mitigating circumstances
7.30am	Home	1 slice of toast and marmite mixed with peanut butter* plus one slice toast with a fried egg	Tea, more tea, water, nurofen	Hangover
11am	work		Diet coke	Bertha says this always works for her
1pm	Café near work	Crisps**	Mineral water	** Bertha says they do the trick too
3pm	work	An apple and some grapes	coffee	Realise not had a vitamin for some time
4-6pm			water	
6.30pm	home	More crisps tuna salad, strawberry yoghurt, banana	water	See earlier Trying to be good now
8.30pm	home		jasmine tea	See above
9pm	home		Small glass cava	Bertha texts to suggest hair of dog
10pm	Home in bed		More jasmine tea	Why do I listen to her?

* NB a combination that sounds iffy but is surprisingly moreish – and very effective as a morning after the night before pick-me-up. As is egg on toast.

** I would concur.

What might we glean from the above? Aside from, in particular case, the fact that too much alcohol is a sure-route to eating all sorts?

What we will be able to see, on a normal week's worth of charts, is the patterns and when the extra calories are going down.

For example, let's say you have a chocolate muffin every day at 11 a.m. Could you have one every other day? And have an apple instead on non-muffin days? If you have crisps every night with a glass of wine (as I generally do) could you make them a treat for Fridays and Saturdays and special occasions, and have something a little less calorific Monday to Thursday?

If you see that you always dip terribly at 4 p.m. and dive into the sweet tea and chocolate biscuits, perhaps you could try a couple of squares of dark chocolate instead – or a piece of cheese – with a coffee?

If you realise you eat quite a lot of bread and carbs in general during your working week – toast and cereal for breakfast as well as a sandwich for lunch – could you resolve to only have protein and vegetables for dinner? At least until the weekends?

It is all about what you can live with. And working round your lifestyle.

If you are at home watching *EastEnders*, you may not mind having some skinless chicken and a salad and drinking water for a night or two. If you're going to a wedding or a birthday party, as we've established, you are going to want to have a glass of champagne and eat pudding. And why not? Why feel miserable? Yes, the books will tell you a way round it – scrape the mayonnaise off your prawns, shake your head to the bread roll – water your fizz down with soda (sacrilege!)

But I say: Go along, enjoy yourself, wear an elasticated waistband if necessary, and make this the week you choose other strategies from this fine tome to make sure you don't end up the size of Milton Keynes. (See section on **Party Weeks**).

Because the only way you are going to be successful in maintaining a normal weight is if you make flab-fighting fit in with your life, not control it.

Strict regimes may be OK if you are a Hollywood star with your own macrobiotic chef and personal trainer. But not for the rest of us ordinary mortals who go to work on the early train, cook for the kids, and whose lunch options generally consist of Tony's Sandwich Bar or Bert's Caff, or trying to remember to grab a couple of biscuits and an apple while packing lunch boxes for the five thousand.

It's not always possible to live on alfalfa shoots and juice of wheat grass, or to knock oneself up a quick acacia berry smoothie when the hunger pangs have kicked in and you're already late for the childminder.

This way of doing things is all about being flexible.

If you find yourself in a week where you are travelling a lot, staying with friends, or stuck at home with a teething baby and the builders in, you may just have to eat what you can get and be forced to eschew your usual exercise.

It's a matter of finding the tricks that work for you and your schedule. And you've got a hundred to choose from.

You may feel that there is nothing massively new and groundbreaking here – perhaps you were already *au fait* with the best ways to curb hunger and the benefits of certain food combinations over others, or the dramatic impact the time of day that you eat or exercise can have on your fat reserves – but it is finding your own unique blend of these tactics that is so effective.

And, you must admit, how undeniably useful it is to now have them all in one handy volume you can keep about your (ever-shrinking) person.

Think of the shelf space you will save when you give all those previously failed Guides to Deprivation to the charity shop.

Depending on which strategies you choose, you may feel a bit hungry sometimes and some of my suggestions may make you feel a tad deprived, but remember the whole beauty of this approach is that nothing is for ever. Read on and you will be in the right mindset to cope with both of them. 'Cos the pay-off is *so* worth it.

Managing your sense of deprivation.

1 Live in the moment, but think of tomorrow.
There's a reason why AA urges its members to take one day at a time. If I tell you that you can never again have fish and chips, you may understandably feel a bit bereft. But if you know you can have battered cod tomorrow, you can manage not to today. Don't look ahead to doing without things, or cutting down, for the next six months. Just employ whatever tactic you've chosen for *today.* You can decide what to do tomorrow when it comes.

2   Have something to look forward to.

Possibly it's tomorrow when you might have the crisps/club sandwich/cherry cheesecake you are not having today.

3   Don't be a wuss.

The world won't end if you don't have much breakfast – you can have a nice lunch. And you'll have forgotten the feeling of missing out on the mid-afternoon biscuits the minute you get this evening's glass of wine in your hand. If you feel deprived remember it is all only temporary – you're going to balance it out later. You're only having a small salad for lunch so you can have a pudding when you go out for dinner this evening. Focus on the passing nature of things and how fantastic you're going to look and feel.

4   Prioritise.

Let us say you routinely eat two slices of toast and marmite for breakfast. Ask yourself this – if you spend an ordinary Tuesday not having toast and marmite, will it be the end of the world? No, it won't – you have months and years of marmite-drenched toast ahead of you. If you spend your best friend's 40th birthday party not allowing yourself champagne and those teeny-tiny portions of fish and chips, which quite frankly, I could eat ten of once the alcohol has hit home, when everyone else is cramming it down like there's no tomorrow, are you going to feel miserable and hard done by? Yes, you probably are and who can blame you. So you do a bit of trading. If the party is on Saturday – you do not tell yourself that your diet starts on Sunday. *No*. You start on Monday. You cut back on the breakfasts – you could have one slice of toast for example – and you eat salad for lunch and you hold firm on the second helping of dinner. You picture yourself on Saturday night, a glass in one hand and a mini burger in the other. You can do without a few nice things to eat in the run up to that fine evening because it's only for a short time and the payoff is going to be *huge*. Namely, you will turn up to the said party with a flatter stomach so will look and feel great, and you can eat all the canapés in sight because you deserve them.

How to deal with hunger.

I First, do not let yourself get so hungry you lose all reason.

Then, remember that unless you are about to fall in a faint and start chewing your own arm (do not ever let yourself get like this!) there is a big difference between being genuinely starving and fancying something to eat. Ask yourself if you really are hungry and not just bored, peckish, or have just walked past a cake shop or seen an advert for Burger King.

Have a glass of water, or a cup of tea. You can live with this feeling for a short while – it's not going to last for ever.

2   Employ visualisation. If you really are hungry, tell yourself those stabbing hunger pains are the feel of fat dissolving from your thighs. Comfort yourself by mentally adding up all the calories your ill-disciplined friends are ramming down their throats. (Or really p*ss everyone off and do it out loud.)

3   Remind yourself you're putting up with hunger now, so you can eat pretty much what you want later, and not put on any weight.

4   Eat something little – a stick of cheese, some dark chocolate, a raw carrot. A little can go a long way if you chew slowly, and drink plenty of water or herbal tea.

5   Tell yourself you can eat some more in one hour: in the meantime, suck a mint, clean your teeth, go do a task, and concentrate on something other than your rumbling stomach. You may get so involved you last longer.

6   Don't be a wuss part two. There are people starving all over the world. You can tolerate no cake for an afternoon.

But there is only any need to feel hungry if that is the kind of tactic you choose – and that won't be every day. The whole point of the Fighting the Flab method is that you find the methods that suits *you*.

You can try one of these tips at a time or try a combination of them – for best results and the admiration and astonishment of your friends as your body is transformed – try to do at least one thing from each flab-fighting section – food and exercise – daily, and consult the dress section as you go.

You might like to speed-read the lot and tick the ones you think might work and scrawl something rude over the ones that fill you with horror. Mix and match, experiment, and remember nothing is for ever. If you decide to cut sugar this week, you can always have a cake fest the next.

No carbs is a really good way to kick start a diet – you'll lose lots. But you could just do that for seven days to give you an incentive to carry on. It won't matter that you're missing bread – you can live with that in the pursuit of a slimmer body, because it's only for this week – next week you can hit that toast again. And maybe cut back the alcohol? Telling yourself that you'll really enjoy that chilled wine at the weekend. With crisps instead of the carrot stick you're looking at now. Hold in your head why you're doing this: because you are going to look and feel fabulous!

Write it here: I am going to look … etc

NB But remember, there are any number of ways to lose weight – haven't we all done it lots of times? The trick is keeping it off – and this is where you need a bit of psychology –

THE POWER OF THOUGHT

An awful lot of weight-control is down to an attitude of mind. I believe that regardless of our current weight we are all either fatties or thinnies at heart.

Answer these six simple questions:

1   Your party guests have gone home and you are looking at a plate of sausage rolls. Do you:
    a) Eat a couple while you're washing up, then cover the rest in cling film to put in the fridge for later.
    b) Give them to the birds.

2   You are staying in a hotel with coffee and tea-making facilities. What do you do with the packet of shortbread biscuits?
    a) Eat it/put it in your handbag or pocket/take it home for the kids.
    b) I'm not sure I've ever noticed any biscuits.

3   You go to an all-you-can-eat buffet. What do you do about pudding?
    a) Have that first in case you don't have room for it when you've worked your way through the 27 savoury options.
    b) Sorry, I don't understand the question.

4 What do you do with your left-over wine?

a) I drink it the next day/I have one of those special suction thingies with which to tightly re-cork it until the following weekend/I freeze it in ice-cube trays to drop into casseroles and sauces.

b) My what?

5 Which of these statements best sums up your work/life balance?

a) Sometimes, when I am very busy, I forget to eat.

b) Sometimes, when I am very busy, I forget friends' birthdays/ my wedding anniversary/my car-keys/to pick up the dry-cleaning/who I am/what day it is.

6 Which of the following statements best sums up your normal diet?

a) I view my body as a highly-complex machine and food as fuel. I therefore try to take in a carefully-calculated allowance of dietary energy, nutritionally balanced to optimise that machine's performance.

b) I get a tad ratty when there's no chocolate.

If you answered:

Mostly a) you are only flicking through this at your fat friend's house while you wait for her to get her zip up.

Mostly b) Me too. This is why we are flab-fighting together.

Yes, basically, we can sum up the two personality types thus:

Fatties save the last sandwich on the plate, Thinnies disdain leftovers, remember.

I am not suggesting that you start being wantonly wasteful – what was cling-film invented for after all? – but you can advance your flab-fighting prowess quite significantly by simply thinking about a slim new you.

Think thin.

There is a lot to be said for the power of positive thinking. Have you noticed how skinny people are always twitching about and never sit still? Tell yourself you are a thin person too and start fidgeting now. Walk briskly instead of waddling along like a fatty, throw the kids' cold chips in the bin instead of hoovering them up (Thinnies disdain leftovers) stand tall, think slimline, and practise an irritating laugh and trilling: *Sometimes you know, I forget to eat altogether* ...

And I'm not entirely joking. Slim begets slim. It's a bit like getting money. In my life, I have been very poor and more comfortably off. When you are poor, nobody wants to give you a bean (unless they fleece you for it). In the old days, if you needed money, you had to go grovelling to the bank manager, trying to pretend you were a responsible individual who could be relied upon to repay your car loan and wouldn't dream of spending the lump sum you were begging for on shoes, Indian takeaways, and finally paying the phone bill before you get cut off, which is exactly how you ran up your last overdraft. He usually said no.

But the moment you temporarily amass a few bob, every financial institution in the land starts chucking it at you – offering to increase your credit limit, give it interest free (until some distance point in the future when they'll slap on a rate of eye-watering proportions), and sending plastic cards through the post you neither want nor asked for.

Somehow, when you are thinner, it is easier to be thinner – your metabolism feels faster, your step springier, you attack life with more joy and oomph, and somehow that rubs off on your innate ability to control your weight. When you are fat you get despondent and slow down. You eat a bit more to try to cheer yourself up, and then you give up and get fatter.

You are going to get slimmer.

My friend, the writer Lynne Hackles (She of the C plan – see Tip No 34) eats puddings with relish – her record, over the course of a five-day writers' conference, was 27 profiteroles. She is not at all fat – in fact she has lost weight in recent years – yet I have never shared a meal with her when she hasn't done dessert. Somebody asked Lynne, as she was tucking into quite a large bowl of hazelnut ice-cream accompanied by a jug of hot chocolate-fudge sauce, how she did it.

"What I do," she said, "is every day, at least once a day, and after huge meals, I stare at myself in the mirror and say, 'I have an amazing metabolism.'"

She does – really. "It is called the power of positive thought," she says simply. "And it works for me."

I have known something similar work for me too. Before I got married, I went on the one big proper diet of my life.

I was mega-committed, counted every calorie obsessively, and was very boring and tedious. I even gave up drinking (it is not a period of my life I want to dwell on).

Every time I wavered, I thought of the wedding photos – determined that if I was going to be in the centre of attention – my all-time favourite place – then it wasn't going to be ruined by wobbly bits poking out of the raw silk.

I also figured I could then eat six hamburgers for lunch once I got on honeymoon and pile it all back on with abandon. Except, oddly, that didn't happen. Well not for quite a while, anyway. I had lost almost a stone and that for months and months, even though I'd gone back to eating normally, with bells on.

We went to the USA – my first visit – and I made the most of the portion sizes. A week later we went to Portugal on a corporate jolly, with the company my husband worked for, and were taken out for an amazing spread of afternoon tea. One of the other women leaned across the table and said, as I stuffed my sixth cake – an exquisite chocolate éclair, I remember – how lucky I was – "to be able to eat all that and still stay so slim". I still feel guilty that I didn't tell her the truth – that I'd worked on it for months and usually I'd be twice the size – but I think now that her words were what helped me keep my weight down.

Because I started to believe them. You could say I stayed at my new low weight because I was busy, I was happy, I was taking lots of exercise. Or you could take the view that I thought I'd finally become the sort of person I'd always envied who could eat and eat and never appear to put on an ounce.

And perhaps because I believed it for a while, it became true …

So tell yourself now:
  I'm going to lose weight.
  I'm going to feel great.
  I shall not feel deprived.
  And if I get hungry?
  I'll get over it …

Ready? Let's cut the theory and get started!

Some of the suggestions in the next part of this book may suit you down to the ground, others may be out of the question (if you have any on-going medical conditions, some may be downright dangerous – check with your doctor first). You might find just one that sings to you and that you stick to through thick and thin and that's terrific. Or you may want to try them all for a day or a week at a time. You've got a hundred to choose from. Some ideas may seem inspired (I hope it's the ones I made up myself) others daft (but remember laughter burns calories and gives the metabolism a boost). And that's OK. Try the ones you fancy, reject the rest, and see what suits. Mix and match and ring the changes. If variety is the spice of life, it is also the key to keeping your weight down.

100 WAYS TO
FIGHT THE FLAB

1 **Eat chocolate.** ('Cos we're being realistic, right?)
I am serious. Although we're talking a few squares, not the
whole supermarket shelf. Dark chocolate is what we're
after. Bloody marvellous stuff. Keep a slab close by at all
times.

I have a bar in the hidden fridge in my writing room and
another in the kitchen. Choose decent quality chocolate –
by this I mean high in cocoa and not overly-processed. Go
for at least 70% cocoa content and preferably 85% (Green
& Black's is good. Bring on the product placement), but any
respectable dark chocolate will bring you all sorts of
benefits.

Before we even mention weight control, dark chocolate
gets the thumbs up. It contains plenty of flavonoids which
have an anti-oxidant effect – i.e. they help protect the body
from those nasty little beasties, free radicals – and the type
that pop up in chocolate are mainly flavanols – the sort that
can help lower blood pressure, and improve blood flow to
the brain and heart. (Flavonols are also found in onions,
kale, broccoli, lettuce, tomatoes, apples, grapes, berries, tea,
and red wine – more of the redoubtable qualities of that little
number later!)

Dark chocolate is also a source of vitamins A, C, B6, and

B12 as well as magnesium, calcium, potassium, copper, and iron. And it gets better. Chocolate contains stearic acid which slows digestion down. This means that a few squares will take a significant edge off your appetite, and leave you feeling fuller for longer. This is where it can come in handy:

When you are hungry between meals – try sucking a couple of squares of dark chocolate slowly. Then wait a bit and see if the hunger abates. You may need to repeat. But even if you end up eating 6 squares, you'll only have taken in 125 calories (I am basing this on Green & Black's 85% dark), and had a relatively low carb, low sugar snack (4.5g of carbohydrate of which 2.7g is sugars).

I promise you it will take you through to lunch or dinner a whole lot better than a bag of crisps or a couple of biscuits, and be more pleasurable than boiled cabbage and a cup of brown rice, all of which would be more calorific. NB I find this is particularly effective if accompanied by a black coffee. I don't drink much of the stuff these days but a cup at my low point of the afternoon (around 4 p.m. when I start feeling peckish and grouchy) – with said chocolate – can then keep me going till it's time to down tools and grab the corkscrew.

In addition, my exhaustive research has revealed that chocolate contains both tryptophan, an essential amino acid that stimulates the production of serotonin – a natural anti-depressant – in the brain, and phenylethylamine, a chemical that stimulates the brain's pleasure centres and creates the sort of feelings we have when in love or having an orgasm (easily confused).

Some claim that phenylethylamine taken as a supplement

works as a weight loss aid and mood enhancer (I am not recommending this – the internet is full of dodgy supplements that don't work and probably give you excess body hair and dizzy spells and I'd never suggest buying anything you're not sure of) while others of a more scientific bent will say that in fact little effect will be experienced if orally ingested.

But I say, as far as the spirit-lifting/aphrodisiac effects of dark chocolate are concerned, the evidence is sufficiently compelling to justify having a few squares to be on the safe side. And my male readers may well see the sense in turning up with a large and exotically packaged box of chocolates under one arm, particularly if hoping to get lucky.

To sum up, very dark chocolate will not only fill you up, but will cheer you up as well (necessary if you've planned to diet and are facing the prospect of cutting out butter and not drinking).

2 Cut out butter and quit drinking.

Now I am joking. Bread without butter is beyond the pale, and as for a plain baked potato ... What you could do if you want to feel virtuous, is to have low-fat cream cheese mixed into your potato instead of the hard stuff – you can jazz it up with chopped onion and/or chives – and swap that glass of wine for a vodka or gin with slimline tonic. A method guaranteed to cut the calories *but* still let you fall over.

3 Eat S-L-O-W-L-Y.

Really do – just take it easy and slow R i g h t D o w n ...
It was Paul McKenna who observed that overweight people
think about food all the time – apart from when they are
actually eating it. Then they are too busy shovelling it down
to actually focus on what they are doing.

It's true – those carrying a surfeit of flab, do usually eat
quickly. And it's the necking it down without thought that
does the damage. If you give your brain a chance to get the
signals from your stomach, it will tell you when to stop.

For example – let us say you feel like some Bournville
chocolate fingers – as I do from time to time. (We are
working with and around our longings and desires aren't
we, so why not?)

After all, a single Cadbury Bournville chocolate finger is
a mere 27.5 calories, 110 for four, the "helping" helpfully
suggested on the packet, so that is not going to break the
calorie bank – as long as you stop there.

If you cram all four in your mouth, crunch and swallow,
you will immediately feel like another four. If you savour
each chocolaty, crunchy mouthful, you will find you get to
the end feeling you've had a real treat and yet you've only
had 110 calories. Result!

How to help yourself slow down.

Aim to chew each mouthful thirty times. This is not easy –
the most I can manage without going mad is about fifteen –
but complete as many mastications as you can.

Drink water with your food. Pause between mouthfuls
and sip.

Listen to soothing music while you eat (I prefer *The Archers*).

Breathe deeply, relax, and repeat unto yourself: if I eat slowly, I will not be such a porker …

4 Learn to Love Chewing!

Research has shown that the longer you chew your food for, the fewer calories you will consume overall. This is not just because you have become bored witless with jaw ache, but because, as tests on volunteers in China revealed, 90 minutes after a marathon chew the levels of Ghrelin (the hormone that gives us our appetite) in one's blood is significantly lower than that of those who have gulped their food down in the manner of a hungry Labrador. So chew, chew, chew – you will feel fuller for longer, and eat less in the whole scheme of things.

5 Think about what you are eating.

Studies have shown that if we are distracted when eating – e.g. we're watching TV at the same time, or have an eye on the clock as we're in a rush, we not only eat more but we also feel hungrier again sooner. Dr Suzanne Higgs, from the University of Birmingham, found indeed that those encouraged to eat slowly and attentively, thinking about each mouthful, were less likely to snack on the post-prandial biscuits offered to them after the meal.

(Unlike, presumably, those bolting their food down with their mind on the iPad in front of them, who were seen necking back the chocolate digestives a mere half hour later.)

6 Take five (or ten, or half an hour).

Carrying on from above, don't only eat slowly but leave gaps in between mouthfuls and portions. If you just wait, before reaching out for some more, you may find you don't need that second helping or third drink, after all.

Remember you need to leave your brain time to catch up with your stomach. Overweight people often eat fast and don't leave that space. And eventually their "I'm full" mechanism becomes so blunted they never do feel properly sated.

Don't end up like that, and if you are there already, start listening to your body and re-educate it.

Have one chocolate cookie or slice of toast and tell yourself, yes you can have another one – in twenty minutes. Go and do something else in the meantime and you may well find you no longer feel the same desperate need to trough it down by then or have become so engrossed you've forgotten you were even going to.

7 Listen to your body!

Years ago, I was very impressed by a book I came across by chance. It was the *Manorama Formula* by Dr M. Legha. The author, a neurologist and scientist, argued that we put on weight because we no longer take note of the natural signals from our bodies. And that if were more in tune with the feelings of being genuinely hungry and then satiated, our bodies would naturally carry the exact amount of fat they were designed to for our height and build.

She described experiments with rats that showed, left to their own devices, they self-regulated, taking in all the nutrients and calories they needed – enough and no more.

And made the point that animals in the wild are never obese because they only eat what their bodies require, as presumably we once did too.

This makes a huge amount of sense to me. I think our bodies know what they need if we can only recognise what they are telling us. Maybe if we want lots of cheese we need the calcium, if we long for a steak we may be tired and low on iron. A fancy for a beautiful chocolate or two, may be our brain wanting the serotonin to lift our low mood.

It is why, perhaps, after eating too much fast food or living on sandwiches, we can suddenly long for fresh vegetables. I can feel positively toxic if I've been burning the candle at both ends and seem to have eaten nothing but toast and canapés for three days. Then I can actively crave a huge salad and turn away willingly from the chocolate biscuits.

NB I have also seen this mechanism at work when bringing up my son.

As a parent, I was a very soft touch about food – nothing was ever forbidden and there were few rules about what could be eaten when.

This was not so much from considerations about health or weight, but because I was a "fussy eater" as a child and the anxiety it caused me lasted years. (The mere phrase "School Dinners" still leaves me in need of a lie-down.)

So when I gave birth to another picky customer, I was determined to accommodate. So what if he had marmite pasta when others ate meat and two veg? Who cared if crisps were high on the menu – they were only potatoes and sunflower oil – or anything green was anathema?

I took the view that contentment came before cabbage,

that no child had actually died from chicken nuggets overload, and that if they came with a vitamin pill, biscuits could make breakfast. And – above all – that time would sort my son's eating habits as, eventually, it sorted mine.

As you might imagine, I was not without my critics: rod-for-your-own-back-blah-blah/five-portions-a-day-or-may-you-burn-in-hell-blah/let no pudding cross his lips before all the meat is eaten, etc.

I ignored them all. I put him off very sugary items – those nasty things they bring back in party bags, with absolutely no food value whatsoever – by referring to them as holes-in-the-teeth-sweets and directing him towards chocolate buttons instead, but I pretty much let him eat anything else.

We had a box with crisps and a tin of biscuits readily available which he could help himself to, and I actually found he would self-regulate.

He could be a pain, like most kids, but he never had a tantrum over anything in the supermarket because food was never an emotional issue. In his teens, our idea of a mother and son bonding session was to declare a fast food day and have a take-away burger for dinner or a pile of fried chicken. So what?

My son still likes his junk food, but he also eats his fruit and veg. But the main point is, despite the protestations of the Food Police, he has grown tall and strong, has only the one head, has passed exams, rarely been to the doctor's, and is normal weight. [1]

Footnote 1 In fairness, he did take lots of exercise too. We sold his buggy as soon as he could walk and my husband once made him cycle five miles to buy a Pokémon card. His therapist will no doubt be informed …

8 Let nothing be forbidden.

If you are listening to your body, then nothing need be. If you want cake, have cake, but a slice, not the entire Victoria sponge – you can have more later or tomorrow. Once we forbid things, we start to crave them. Hence on day one of your carb-free diet you will start fantasising about crumpets, even if you haven't eaten one for three years. Tell yourself you can have anything at all you like – any time – but you will need to balance it out. If you have cake for breakfast, then it's a raw tomato for lunch. Think of it as robbing Peter to make sure Paul doesn't end up with a gastric band.

9 Eat when you're hungry, stop when you're not.

This sounds simple, but for various reasons, some of which have been outlined above, we often carry on eating long after we need to. It could be, as previously stated, that we've stopped listening to our signals, or it might be that we were brought up to finish our plates and leaving food is deeply ingrained as a no-no. We may be afraid of appearing ungrateful or unappreciative if someone else has done the cooking, or want to be one of the crowd if everyone else around the table is still stuffing if down. Or we may have a thing about "waste".

Or we may simply carry on eating because whatever we have on our plates tastes really nice and we're getting pleasure from that, and we're going to feel like we're missing out if we leave the rest of it. If we even pause to analyse it at all – it's more likely we won't give what we are doing a thought, but just carry on stuffing it in!

But if we can learn to only eat when we actually need to

– whether we then choose to eat an orange or a muffin – we can eat what we fancy and never be overweight.

How do we do this?

Eat slowly.

Take lots of pauses between mouthfuls.

Stop and consciously ask yourself – do I really need any more?

And if you're at home, put a plate over the rest and stick it in the fridge – you can always have it later or tomorrow.

Remember that if your body doesn't need this food it is going to be wasted anyway, by being stored as fat or passing back out again.

If you've been cooked for, a charming smile – and the right words about how delicious it was, but so filling … won't lose you friends.

And if you don't want to stick out from the crowd in a restaurant you can always play with it till everyone else has finished.

As for missing out? Will you remember tomorrow how you felt when you didn't eat the last seven chips? What you'll be feeling tomorrow is flatter-stomached, more energised, and proud of yourself. Anyone can clear a plate …

10 Embrace the freezer as your friend.

Leftovers are great but they are also a huge temptation to eat more than you really want to. So freeze them – while you're still full from dinner – rather than always putting them in the fridge. Then you won't see them so readily and it will be more of a faff – as they'll need to be got out and defrosted – to eat them.

This will give you valuable time for reflection on whether you *really* want to gobble down last night's pasta, before you go to bed/for breakfast, when either a nice cup of green tea with lemon and a brisk walk round the block/scrambled egg and well-grilled bacon would be so much more beneficial in boosting your metabolism/setting you up for the day. NB if you haven't got a freezer, pack leftovers up in foil so you can't see the contents and put them at the back of the fridge – anything to make them harder to get at.

11 Bake but don't binge.

The freezer is also a godsend when you have the urge to bake. Baking is lovely and therapeutic and immensely satisfying. But can also lead to massive overeating just because the end product smells so good and is moreish.

So have one slice of cake and hand it round, then freeze the rest rather than putting it in a tin, where it's oh-so-accessible. If you cut it up first you can defrost one portion at a time and other family members can do likewise.

I like making bread because I find it soothing and it makes the house smell delicious, and I know exactly what's in it (only flour, water, yeast, salt, a pinch of sugar, and a splash of olive oil – no rubbish or additives or so much sugar you can taste it).

I make batches of rolls – with my hands, not a machine – and freeze all but the few we want immediately as soon as they are cool. Thus removing temptation and the tendency to say: I'd better have my third, you know, or they'll all go stale …

12 A chilli a day keeps a fat arse at bay.

So eat a chilli. The hotter the better. Chillies raise the metabolism and the more fiery they are, the greater the effect. Experts estimate that one can expect a 15% increase in calories burned for about two hours after eating a hot chilli sauce. Buy packets of fresh chillies from the supermarket and then keep and dry the seeds. Growing them yourself is (without wishing to sound like an excerpt from *Cooking on a Shoestring in a Bedsit for One*) easy, cheap, and satisfying and the plants look pretty on the kitchen window sill (you can see a photo of mine – as well as the chilli-infused olive oil I bottle when I was last being a domestic goddess (ha!) – on the Fight the Flab blog www.100waystofighttheflab.com. [2]

Try them finely chopped in omelettes and scrambled egg, over meat or fish, in sauces and – for the brave – straight down with a couple of crisps. Actually you will find the more you eat, the more your tolerance will grow (I don't wish to be indelicate here, but it is best to build up slowly!) They are strangely addictive after a while. Now I begin to twitch if I don't have my regular fix.

13 Don't eat in the evenings.

The earlier you stop eating, the more food you'll get away with. The theory is that if you don't eat after late afternoon, your body has all evening to burn up what you *have* eaten. Whereas if you turn in at midnight after three jam sponges

Footnote 2 This also contains photos of my bottom. Don't say you weren't warned

and a lard sandwich, you have all night for your body to convert that into another layer of blubber across your middle. I can eat any amount of breakfast and lunch as long as I stop then, and don't have anything else but water or green tea. Have a go yourself. If I take in no calories after about 4pm I'll always wake up with the scales unaltered or even showing a loss. This is clearly not always practical, but do avoid eating too late.

14 Walk before bed.

This should really be in the exercise section, but this tip works so brilliantly, that I wanted you to read it as soon as possible so you could try it. I am almost evangelical about this one because I know beyond doubt that it allows me to eat lots more than I would otherwise dare. A brisk march round the block before you hit the sack will boost your metabolism no end and help burn off whatever you've been stuffing in front of *Newsnight*. To put it to the test, eat the same as usual but do this for a week. You'll be surprised how much thinner you feel. NB if you live somewhere dodgy you might want to take a large partner or friend with you. If he or she is very large you will feel thinner anyway.

15 Do *something* before bed.

For those of you already mounting objections e.g. I live in a high rise flat on the edge of a motorway; I live in a place where you don't walk to the corner in broad daylight let alone round the block at night; I have small children and no babysitter, my dog is afraid of the dark; then for you and only for you (the rest of you, just shift yourselves and try it) do some kind of exercise at home before you go to bed. This might include: running up and down the stairs, doing some sit ups, watching *News at Ten* sitting on an inflatable ball (see exercise section proper), jogging on the spot, scrubbing the kitchen floor, taking the rubbish out, engaging in a spot of DIY, or doing some vigorous ironing. (NB the latter has the additional advantage of getting you brownie points for being a domestic god/goddess and the chance to hold forth on how you were immersed in domestic drudgery while the rest of the family were vegged out on the sofa.)

16 Cut out sugar.

First they came for the smokers, then the drinkers were taken to task, now the latest in the firing line for doing Things that are Bad for You are the sugar eaters.

There are calls to tax sugary drinks in the UK and some supermarkets already "red light" products high in fructose. Quite aside from what it can do to your teeth and waistline, high sugar consumption is now linked to type 2 diabetes, high blood pressure, liver problems, heart disease, kidney disease, a depressed immune system, and ropey skin. And I must say, even to me, who gets wearied and cynical about the constant barrage of doom-mongering about anything that is vaguely enjoyable, the evidence is compelling.

Having read about the work of Robert Lustig (*Fat Chance: The Bitter Truth about Sugar*. Fourth Estate. You can also see him on YouTube) and David Gillespie (*The Sweet Poison Quit Plan*. Penguin) it makes perfect sense to me that sugar can become as addictive as alcohol or cigarettes. And I haven't drunk fruit juice since.

Not all scientists agree on the finer details, but research from all directions confirms that it tends to be sugar, not fat, that is responsible for the obesity epidemic and all sorts of other nasties on top. You may not believe you can possibly be eating the amount of sugar claimed as the average – anything up to 140 teaspoonfuls per week, depending on who you read – the latter was from the National Diet and Nutrition Survey for the NHS – but you might be surprised.

Particularly invidious are the hidden sugars lurking in everything from bread to "low-fat" salad dressings and even popping up where you'd least expect them – balsamic vinegar has 12-15% of the sweet stuff – who knew? It is the fructose element to sugar – widely used as a commercial sweetener – that does the damage.

Fructose, the research tells us, goes straight to the liver to be processed as fat, yet isn't registered by the brain as containing calories, and therefore does not switch on our appetite-control mechanism.

Those who go about drastically cutting sugar from their diets report an increase in energy and vitality, fewer mood swings and clearer skin, as well as weight loss. If you eat a great deal of it to start with, you are likely to suffer withdrawal symptoms – headaches, grumpiness, even the jitters, but David Gillespie reports losing six stone, even though he made no other changes to his lifestyle. It might be worth a go!

How to reduce your sugar consumption:

Read the labels – you'll be amazed what's got sugar in it.

Cut out fizzy drinks, concentrated fruit juice, jams, sweet

spreads, chutneys, and sugary breakfast cereals, as well as the obvious cakes, biscuits, and sweets.

Or if this is too drastic, try to spend a little time each shopping trip on searching out the brands or products that have a lower sugar content. For example, shortbread fingers generally contain less sugar than dried fruit bars! And there's less sugar in a Cadbury's dark chocolate finger than a Wagon Wheel.

If baking at home, use a third or even half the usual amount of sugar. I bet you, or anyone else eating the results, won't really notice the difference.

Gin, vodka, or dry white wine are lower sugar options compared to sweet wines or liqueurs, beer or cider. Use slimline mixers.

NB I was recently given a totally delicious sugar-free chocolate by Victoria and Brendan, who run the Cocoa Exchange, (www.thecocoaexchange.com), and use malt extract as a sweetener for their diabetic range. Their general ethos is very low sugar and they offer chocolate that has a 90% cocoa solid and "a grain reminiscent of old fashioned chocolate from years ago that lasts longer on the tongue with a slower melting point in the mouth". Victoria tells me that their gourmet chocolate is all about eating a little bit at a time, savouring it with great enjoyment and being left satisfied rather than craving more. I am going to investigate further!

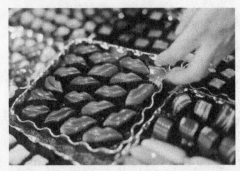

Chocolates from the Cocoa Exchange Range

17 Eat fruit, instead of drinking smoothies.

Smoothies can have more sugar and calories in them than cola! If you eat the actual fruit, you munch on all the fibre too, which slows down the absorption of sugar into the system and gives the liver a chance to cope. There is also the theory, mentioned earlier, that the actual process of chewing helps you feel full too – so whereas a glass of apple juice will go straight down in an instant and have no effect on your hunger levels except to give you a sugar rush, eating a whole apple will properly count to your body as food and may take the edge off your appetite.

NB excessive consumption of fruit juice is none too kind to the enamel on your teeth either.

18 Declare a junk-free day each week.

If the above is all too scary – just try it for one day each week. Declare a day of virtue and try really hard, just for 24 hours, to cut out sugar, eat no processed or junk food, grill and bake, rather than deep fry, and drink water rather than alcohol.

61

At the very least you will wake up brighter of eye and with an extra zing, and you can hardly fail to eat fewer calories. Yes, you may find it dull, and think wistfully of crisps, but it's only till tomorrow.

19 Only eat with a knife and fork.

This was my son Tom's contribution as a diet tip – and I must say it's quite a good one. There are two variations on it.

The basic idea is that you eat nothing that you'd naturally eat with your fingers – so no crisps, biscuits, chocolates, peanuts, sandwiches, hamburgers (I said it was his tip, not that he'd actually tried it), no fruit indeed. Try it for a day – you'll find yourself having to eat "proper meals" and pretty good stuff at that. The alternative is to eat what you like but you *must* use a knife and fork, regardless of what it is you're having (tried eating crisps or bar of fruit and nut like that?). At the very least, it will slow you down.

20 Do weigh yourself if you want to.

The received wisdom is often to only weigh yourself once a week or so, but the problem with this is that if you happen to hit on a day when for any number of reasons, your weight is up by a pound or two, it can be terribly dispiriting.

Better, I think, to weigh yourself every day if you want to (though do it at the same time each day – preferably first thing in the morning, with no clothes on, after you've had your first pee and before you've eaten or drunk anything) but bear in mind the likely fluctuations and look at the overall picture rather than the daily reading. It really doesn't matter if your weight goes like this (I am a dinosaur and still prefer my weight in old money rather than kilos):

Monday: X Stone, 5lb

Tuesday: X Stone, 4lb

Wednesday: X Stone, 6lb

Thursday: X Stone, 5lb

Friday: X Stone, 4lb

Saturday: X Stone, 5lb

Sunday: X Stone, 4lb

Monday: X Stone, 3lb

As long as the overall result is that you weigh the same or less (depending on what your aim is) this week as/than you did last. The problem with the once-a-week method is that nobody can bear to wait a week, so you cave in on Saturday – the night after you had a curry on Friday (always guaranteed to up the weight – something to do with spicy food and fluid retention), find you haven't lost anything or, worse, if you only lasted till the Wednesday on our particular chart, you've actually put it on.

Then you get thoroughly disheartened, convince yourself you are destined to be hefty for ever and eat everything in the biscuit cupboard to drown your sorrows because you might as well. When all the time you were doing OK after all. So if you're going to be a slave to the scales, be a proper one. Weigh daily, keep a record, and take an average. *Or* give the machine to the charity shop and:

21 Use a tape measure.

The tape cannot lie. Everyone knows that muscle does weigh more than fat and that weight can fluctuate wildly all on its own (try getting up and weighing yourself, walking round a bit, drinking half a cup of herbal tea, and weighing yourself again. You've had no calories, a pint of water weighs a pound and a quarter and you've only had 300 mls, and you've suddenly put on a pound and a half! How?).

The tape measure will tell it as it is and will demonstrate conclusively whether your girth has increased overnight or you took my advice and sprinted down the road and back. As will a "measuring skirt" or pair of trousers. Pick something you can only wear on thin days and try it on. If the zip does up you're doing fine whatever the scales say. If your stomach is bulging through the gap like an uncooked suet pudding, it's time to hit the hot water with lemon and ginger.

22 Drink hot water with lemon and ginger.

Apparently hot water makes your stomach feel full, lemon juice takes the edge off your hunger, and ginger boosts the metabolism. I can't vouch for this. I just know it doesn't sound as nice as a glass of Macon Blanc Villages and a bag of Kettle Chips.

23 Cut the carbs.

There is no doubt about it, however much you may be clinging on to that packet of custard creams, that this works. Eat no rice, potatoes, bread, cakes, pasta, etc. and you will lose weight. And the benefit of the high protein approach –

lots of meat, fish, eggs, cheese, with salad or vegetables – is that if you do it properly you won't feel hungry either. (Bored and deprived possibly, but certainly not starving.)

In fact, after a while, as you rediscover your hip bones and note just the one chin looking back at you, you may find you really feel quite energised and jolly. I think it's the smug feeling of virtue that cheers me up!

Opponents of this plan, usually to be identified by the plate of chips in their hands, will whine on about heart disease and cholesterol levels but really they're just feeling bitter about the lack of biscuits.

This is my diet plan of choice if I am going to focus on losing a few pounds for a special event. I don't do it as strictly as the Atkins, in that I have unlimited salad and veg from the start (no fruit), or in such a complex way as the Dukan (oh dear have you noticed the way all the really multi-million-pound-whole-industry-potential mega-best-selling diet books are two syllables? Atkins, Dukan, Five:two? Is the Wenham-Jones going to cut it? The *100 Ways to Fight the Flab* certainly isn't – that's a whole bloody eight. If you can reduce it down to two syllables for the reprint, please get in touch) – which involves little dairy and some oatbran stuff and only fat-free fromage frais but I do something I think of as "Atkins plus wine and peanuts" which follows the basic principle and works.

On it I'm allowed:

Any fish or meat.

Eggs and vegetable proteins like quorn.

Any cheese.

Nuts and seeds.

Avocados and tomatoes (strictly fruits but I treat them as a vegetable for this purpose).

Should I want it: plain yoghurt, fromage frais, cream (though I don't tend to eat much of this and I hate plain milk so would only include this if making a cheese sauce), wine and dark chocolate (though I try to switch to gin and slimline tonic for some of the duration).

I forbid myself all the carb-heavy stuff and limit fruit to an occasional pick at it.

I feel quite happy eating avocados and prawns with mayo, and Caesar salads (hold the croutons) or big cheese and ham omelettes, so it suits me. And the thing about the high protein/low carb approach is that you will definitely not be hungry. In fact, I frequently can't get to the end of the mega salads (see more of them later) I make when on such a regime. And if you want to be obsessive about it (it's the only way I can manage sometimes), you can buy Ketostix – little plastic testing strips to keep in the loo to pee on, with which to check you are in ketosis – which you will be if you don't eat carbs.

This is rather satisfying as it means you know your body is burning up fat – and as long as you have no underlying health problems, this is perfectly fine in the short term as long as you drink lots of water.

What I also like about the low carbohydrate approach is that I can hold a simple mantra in my head.

Eating Fat and Protein promotes Fat Burning.

Eating Carbs promotes Fat Storage.

I remind myself of this when I'm starting to hyperventilate

about wanting toast. I also remind myself nothing is forever, and once I have got into the dress/turned up at the big bash/had my photo taken, I can go get a baguette.

Verdict: Useful for a quick fix when you've got two weeks to get into the dress you haven't done up since 2006.

24 Cut some of your carbs or eat them early.

If the above is too strict, or you are interested in maintaining your weight rather than losing shedloads of it, just follow the low-carb approach for one meal a day. You will be amazed at how effective this will be whenever you do it, but for maximum effect have no carbs in the evenings. Have your porridge or muffin for breakfast and your sandwich or baked potato for lunch, or your mid-afternoon bun, but in the evening stick to protein and veg or salad and have fruit rather than jam roly-poly. No need to feel hard done by because you can eat what you like, just have it early.

25 Only eat carbs for an hour.

This is very roughly the method propounded upon in *The Carbohydrate Addict's Diet* by Dr Rachel Heller and Dr Richard Heller (Vermilion). The idea is that you only eat carbohydrates/all the stuff you really want to eat, within a one hour window each day.

Other meals are low carb/sugarless – e.g. grilled chicken and a green salad or scrambled eggs and bacon. You can have alcohol but again, within that hour.

I really liked the idea of this when I read about it but I couldn't make it work for me. If I'm going to have lovely stuff to eat, I like to have a glass of wine while I'm getting it all together and then eat in a leisurely fashion. If I go out to lunch with friends I want to linger over it. And eat the chocolate mint with my coffee.

It sounds a long time, but an hour seems to flash by when you know you've got to cease eating on the dot. And you do have to be precise for the science of this diet to work. But others rave about it so you might too. Get the book, read the theory, and give it a go!

26 Cut the fat.

Doing this is much, much worse. You are condemning yourself to a dreary existence of dry toast, flavourless leaves, bad-temper and hunger (or was that just me?). Yes a multi-million pound fortune may have been built on the premise that if you give up butter you'll get thinner legs but if you're that desperate to lose ten pounds it is probably less painful to cut a leg off.

27 When eating fat, stick to the "good" stuff.

Slather on the butter by all means – it's a wholefood. Splash on the olive oil – it's full of essential fatty acids omega 3 and 6, potatoes roasted in goose fat – similar make-up to olive oil – why not?

But a dodgy looking pie of questionable provenance full of hydrogenated fats and very probably animal bottoms, toenails and upper lips? Personally I wouldn't.

28 Know what's in it, if not bin it.

If I had a mantra for healthy-eating, this would be it: see above! If you had one absolute rule and that was that you only ate things you could guarantee all the ingredients of, i.e. you'd made it yourself or had a good look at the packaging and knew there were no saturated fats, fructose, hydrogenated nastiness, or strange numbers lurking within, and that was the only rule you followed, I bet you a bottle of extra virgin to a pound of lard – you'd lose weight.

29 Cut the wheat and dairy.

Nobody is anybody these days unless they have a food intolerance. Obviously, if you swell up and die when you see a peanut, you have my sympathy, and I myself must admit to a small tendency to get stomach ache if I eat much meat. But on the whole, let's face it, the whole thing's become a bit of a nonsense. If God had wanted us to eschew bread and butter, why would he have invented the egg mayonnaise sandwich? But when one day, some years ago, one of my friends announced she'd "simply given up wheat and dairy" and was suddenly swanning about looking at least a stone lighter with perfect skin, that was galling. And there is always something seductive about the quick fix. The idea that one might revolutionise one's entire life and looks by cutting out one ingredient had to be worth a try. It wasn't as if you had to do it for ever. I figured you could give up pizza for a month when you needed to look gorgeous for some big event and then capitulate later when it was all over and it didn't matter if you were fat and blotchy. So I tried no wheat or dairy, myself. It was very boring. And since it meant I couldn't stuff down the bread in restaurants while I was waiting, I used to get very drunk. I went to a long lunch – it might have been a Romantic Novelists' Association

Awards ceremony, where the entire menu – all cheese sauce, crêpes, and filo pastry shapes – featured something I couldn't eat. In three hours I had a tomato, three green beans, and two bottles of burgundy. My friend, the writer Lynne Barrett-Lee, who had to pour me into a cab when I could no longer speak, said if I ever did it again she would wrestle me to the floor and ram a roll down my throat.

30 Give up yeast.

This advice was delivered, sternly, by a Thin Friend looking hard at my fat stomach. "It will sort your bloating," she said. I will tell you what sorted my bloating – it was having a hysterectomy. This may be a bit drastic for you (especially if you're one of my male readers) but if you were considering one anyway, I can confirm that a flatter abdomen afterwards was one of the better by-products. (Being pumped full of HRT instead of flinging the crockery about for half the month was another. But that's a different book[3].) I was mildly tempted to ban yeast until I met the TF's colleague who had. We shall call her Ursula Uptight. She claimed she'd been blood-tested, yeast was the culprit, and it was never going to pass her lips again. When I saw her she'd lost loads of weight and looked a million dollars. But you wouldn't want to go out with her. In the restaurant she barged her way into the kitchen to root through the ingredients on every packet and jar, wouldn't have mayonnaise or drink wine, and sat in front of an empty plate all night with a face on. This put me off the whole idea.

Footnote 3 see my fourth novel PRIME TIME.

Apparently there is yeast in everything. Weight loss through starving yourself is a recognised method already and how was I supposed to cope without Marmite? (Don't forget it's good for a hangover, mixed with peanut butter.) But under the joint pressure of the born-again intolerants, I sent off for the test they'd taken – a "simple pin-prick blood test" which was quite scientific-looking and involved a small, round plastic thing that you clicked onto your thumb. Being both of a squeamish nature and a wimp, I asked a friend to perform the necessary. "Press down firmly" he read aloud as he pressed and I screamed. Investigation inside the plastic thing showed something resembling half a Stanley knife. I bled for five minutes. There was plenty to dip the stick in anyway and I packed it off waited for the outcome, dreaming fondly of finding out I was intolerant to something like lentils or semolina that I didn't think much of anyway and shedding half of my body weight overnight; and vowing not to tell anyone if it turned out to be red wine or crisps. It turned out to be nothing at all. Test Result Negative, said the letter, rather disappointingly, from the Medical Director. Said it was a nonsense.

31 Cut everything and eat yoghurt and banana.

This idea came from my friend Irene who swears by this unlikely-sounding regime which has one simple rule – you can eat as much as you like of absolutely anything as long as it is plain yoghurt or banana. You are supposed to do it for three days. Since banana is a diuretic and yoghurt an evacuant (let's not go there) it does work, but by dawn of the second day you are out of your head with the tedium of it and are hallucinating about toast and marmite or anything that isn't bloody yogurt or banana. Not unlike the Squeeze-into-Trousers-too-Small Plan which involves:

32 Grapes.

By this method you eat nothing but grapes for as long as it takes till you can do your party togs up. Purists say that that you should eat the skins and stalks and pips (fibre, I believe!) and offer the helpful advice that you should persevere through the nausea and headaches (toxins clearing, don't you know) and vary the mind-numbing monotony by sometimes making a grape smoothie (but you know what we've already said about them!). Oh and you can drink lots of water too – hot OR cold, just to add to the excitement. I have no doubt you will lose weight if you try this – you may also feel like jumping off the nearest bridge. As I have already indicated, the only time I attempted it when wishing to wear a slinky black dress without looking like a black pudding, I lasted three hours. Try small squares of dark chocolate instead (see point one).

33 Try intermittent fasting.

This, as you will know, is all the rage. Devotees (backed up by some reasonable science) swear that arranging your life into "feed" and "fast" days will not only keep your weight down but help you live longer. I first read about the benefits of fasting in an article by Amanda Ursell for the *Sunday Times Style* magazine back in 2005. She spoke of research that suggested that alternate feasting and fasting did not suppress the metabolism the way traditional calorie-cutting did and recommended a day of eating only a 360 calorie meal followed by a day of eating what you like, before going back to the "fast" again, and so on.

In 2012 the medical journalist, Michael Moseley, experimented with a similar scheme in which he ate only 500 calories on two days of the week for the BBC's TV programme *Horizon* and since then, and the publication of his best-selling book, *The Fast Diet*, everyone is at it. A raft of celebrities are followers of what has become popularised as the 5:2 and you can hardly walk to the corner shop without bumping into someone who's taking up a lot less of the pavement than they used to. If you hand your box of chocolates round the office, at least one of your colleagues will wave it away with a "I'm on a fast day" and possibly a slightly haunted expression.

The method goes roughly like this: you eat normally (whatever you like, they say!) on five days of the week and then on the other two (non-consecutive) days – say Monday and Thursday – you eat either nothing at all (if you are totally obsessed with this theory and probably American) or you just have 500 calories (if you're not). The effectiveness of the diet is down to the activation of a the SIRT1 gene (also known as the "Skinny Gene" which is involved in cell repair and maintenance and has been shown to inhibit fat storage and have anti-ageing benefits.

When I first heard about it I couldn't wait to try it. The thought of losing weight and controlling the crow's feet was irresistible. It appealed to me psychologically because a) you can stand pretty much anything if it only lasts 24 hours b) I do love a quick fix c) the thought of being able to stuff burgers and chips with abandon for the rest of the week was a good one.

AND I read an interview with one chap (in America) who does it and who is super healthy and slim (with lovely American teeth) and he didn't even starve for what we consider a day. He went from 2 p.m. to 2 p.m. which frankly anyone should be able to do. I tried from 6 p.m. to 6 p.m. on the basis that when I came out of my non-eating phase I would be able to celebrate with a glass of cava with my chips.

This was my report at the time:

It does work – I lost a pound in the short term – but you would have to do it *every* week. And whatever two days you designate for not eating are guaranteed to be the days you are invited out for breakfast, lunch, and afternoon tea and then someone suggests a take-away. (My friend, the novelist Katie Fforde, said for her, it would have to be re-named the Procrastination Diet.)

Since then, I cannot claim to have carried out much more exhaustive formal research than that – I have probably enjoyed approximately 359 feast days to 6 fast – but, as you will have gathered, I utterly believe in the principles of feast and famine balancing out.

Eat the canapés at the party with gusto – if you can manage to balance a glass in one hand, a cocktail stick, napkin, and mini salmon fishcake in the other, dunk said cocktail snack in the dip without it dripping down your front, and still keep up a thrilling conversation – but don't then go out for a massive dinner afterwards.

If you want afternoon tea, with scones, and jam, and little

triangular sandwiches as well as several cakes, then do have it, by all means, but make this your big pig-out of the day and do not expect to do lunch and supper as well and come out of it the same size.

Sometimes I do a 5:2 – more of a six-one really – thing by default. I get busy or am moving about and haven't been able to eat. I don't mean I'm one of those annoying people who "forgets" but I get involved, or I'm on a train with no buffet car and suddenly realise I have a hunger pain and it's 3pm and all I've had is a digestive biscuit since the night before.

At that point I might do a quick calculation and think: ah ha – if I can hold on until 8 p.m., I'll have done twenty-four hours, so I'll make a conscious effort to eat as little as possible – if not abstain altogether until the appointed time arrives.

I don't know conclusively if this helps keep my weight stable – it probably does – but I don't think it's too difficult to survive for a day on only five hundred calories, especially if you know the world is your culinary oyster on the next. And I know several people who have lost shedloads of fat on the plan. Betty Orme, who I met at the fabulous Chez-Castillon, in the Dordogne in France where I teach on writing courses a couple of times a year, has been doing the 5:2 for the last nine months and has visibly shrunk a bit more each time I've seen her.

Betty, "76-years-young", began the diet because her increased weight had started, as she puts it, "to take its toll" on her knee joints and she was into what she describes as a "a vicious circle; obesity making exercise impossible without pain." Betty had read about the 5:2 diet and knew someone who'd lost weight on it. She'd been given a treadmill by friends who no longer had the space for it, and when the New Year came around made a resolution to start the 5:2 and combine with it with daily exercise on the treadmill until she was 25kgs lighter (a fair old undertaking – I think I am marvellous if I lose 3kg).

Betty usually has her fasting days on Tuesday and Friday, drinking water or black coffee and eating only a salmon fillet, cooked in the microwave, in a mixture of a little lemon juice, pepper and butter, with salad or spinach, or other vegetable, followed by a yoghurt or piece of fruit, and is strict about keeping to her 500 calories on these two days.

"I find it much easier if I make sure that I am really busy," she says, "so that I have no time to think about food."

On the other 5 days, she eats "more or less what I fancy" – and she likes a glass of wine or a G & T – although she says she often finds she now automatically eats "very sensibly" even on feast days. As I write, Betty has lost 18 kgs and intends to lose the final 7kg over the next 4 months.

Writer Kate Harrison, who I met through the Romantic Novelists' Association, is in her forties and had been dieting for all her adult life when she discovered the approach, which, she says, has changed her life.

"It has absolutely revolutionised my weight and my approach to eating. On previous diets – low-carb, for example – I'd get to my ideal weight but then want to eat the 'banned foods' again and as soon as I had even a bit of toast, the guilt would make me feel I'd failed. Intermittent fasting is so simple."

Kate has now lost 28lbs and dropped from a UK size 14/16 to a 10/12. She looks, I have to say, stunning! She intends to stick to the plan for life both for the weight control and the health benefits.

"There's lots of cancer in my family, and type 2 diabetes, and the potential to cut my risk of those is a great motivator," she says. Kate set up her own Facebook group for a few friends who were trying the regime. At the time of writing, it now has 12,500 members, and Kate, who has since become the author of *The 5:2 Diet Book* and *The Ultimate 5:2 Recipe Book* has taken the principles even further. Her third title in the series is *5:2 Your Life,* in which she applies the theory to work, fitness, and even your love life! (Which can also of course be a fine weapon in the Flab-fighting armoury – see Tip No. 84 ☺.)

But the 5:2 has its detractors – some complain that the fasting days leave dieters tired and unproductive and lead them to binge the moment they are allowed to start eating again.

And as we know, there is always a fresh diet just around the corner. The very latest twist on the intermittent fasting front comes from Patrick Holford with *Burn Fat Fast: The alternate-day low-GL diet plan* – a diet of low GL (Glycaemic Load) which as far as I can see is the same as low GI (foods low on the Glycaemic index) and offers its own take on fasting – you eat 800 calories for three days a week – or every other day basically, rather than 500 calories for two, but you eat these low GL, slow release foods, chosen to manage your insulin levels, burn off your fat, and also play an anti-ageing role.

Whatever the maths, to me it stands to reason that if overall you are consuming less food and fewer calories, you are going to lose weight and if this helps keeps the old wrinkles and saggy bits at bay too, so much the better. Balancing your feed-your-face instincts with a little restraint is what Fighting the Flab is all about too.

So if you've been good all day, go have a chocolate. ☺

34 Follow the C Plan.

My friend, the aforementioned writer Lynne (a surprising number of my friends have this name) Hackles conceived this. And it is ingenious. The rules are simple. You can eat anything you like as long as it doesn't begin with that letter. So no Cream, Chocolate, Chips, Crisps, Cake etc. It sounds really good. But it doesn't work. Especially if you pig out on Gateau and French Fries.

35 Pick a letter of the alphabet and make a plan of your own.

I have been trying to think of an initial letter that encompasses all good stuff and that if you stuffed that all day long you wouldn't put on weight. T was looking hopeful – tuna, tomatoes, trout, turkey, tangerines, turnips, tofu, tahini paste – until I remembered trifle, treacle and tiramisu, and S – Strawberries, salad, sardines, salmon, sunflower seeds, and spinach – falls down badly when you hit the sherry with your sandwiches, sausage rolls, suet, and syllabub. So far A is heading the pack – almonds, arugula, Allspice, anchovies, avocados, asparagus, apples, aubergine, apricots, and artichokes, should fill you with health and vitality unless you start making pies and crumbles with the apples and suddenly remember Aero bars and After Eights. Although even then, you should get away with the sweet stuff after all that fruit and veg.

Try it yourself for a fun way to limit your range of foodstuffs for a day or a week (better take a vitamin pill if you're living on wine, waffles, and Worcestershire sauce). Let me know if any one letter actually works for you ...

You can make your own list here:

Letter	Letter	Letter	Letter

36 Have short-term goals.

If your aim is to lose weight then short-term goals can be very useful to keep you focussed. "I am going to lose two stone in six months" can feel daunting but – "I am going to look much better in two weeks' time" is far more manageable. Hold a date in mind – a party or a holiday or visiting friends you haven't seen for a while – and use the vision of you looking slimmer and fitter on this occasion, to help you stay motivated.

Brides usually manage to lose weight for their big day because the thought of bulging out of one's wedding dress and having to look at the photos for ever more is a much more dismal prospect than skipping dinner.

So think of a short-term reason for really working hard at your weight loss. Comfort yourself with the thought that after that, you can have a feast, but for now you are going to just reach the appointed weekend and look fab at that birthday celebration or wow them at the school reunion. Then, when you've got there and floated off on all the compliments, you can set another goal.

For real motivation there is nothing like knowing you have to wear a particular outfit and that if you don't lose weight, it will look terrible, or even that you won't actually get it on at all! In fact I am tempted to suggest buying a dress or trousers on the tight side, prior to a big do, to force yourself to slim down. It has worked for me. But before I encourage you to follow suit, I should offer this cautionary tale.

For the last few years I have wielded the microphone at the RoNas (The Romantic Novel of the Year awards) and have fallen into the habit of donning a somewhat over-the-top frock. I've worn a full length fuchsia-pink glittery number a sparkly silver job and most recently a gown in midnight blue with "embellishments". I think the main embellishment was in the sizing, which, judging from the struggle I had to pull up the back zip, was clearly cut on the small side. But it's a faff returning things on the internet and I did like the look of it, so I told myself that a bit of flab lost would make all the difference.

But just to make sure, I put it on back to front, did up both zip and hook and eye, eased it the right way round and then hoisted it up over my bosom and managed to squeeze my arms into place.

I couldn't breathe or sit down and the general effect was pantomime milkmaid, but I could see that with a few pounds gone – and confident in the knowledge that with my own flab-busting tips to follow this was perfectly achievable in the time frame – it would fit the bill.

I twirled a couple of times in front of the mirror, wondered idly about where one would find midnight blue shoes, made a mental note to do lots of sit-ups – it was extremely tight across my middle – and decided to keep it. Then I tried to take it off.

With my arms pinned in the sleeves, it was impossible to reach behind me to undo the back, I couldn't get my arms free to get it over my head and, thus trapped, I couldn't wriggle it round again to release the hook and eye. I was alone in the house – my husband not due back for some hours, the boy for a couple of days – and was soon trying not to hyperventilate while reassuring myself that it really wasn't tight enough to cut off my entire blood supply.

Before real panic set in, I spotted a delivery man coming up the path. I waddled down the stairs as fast as one can when in the equivalent of a straitjacket, intending to explain the situation and ask if he'd mind doing a spot of unhooking, hoping if the request were made with enough cheer and jollity he wouldn't think me some sort of desperate housewife. (I have never forgotten the expression on the face of the meter reader when I opened the door unaware that all my shirt buttons were undone.)

I threw open the door but before I could draw breath, he'd taken one startled look, dumped the parcel, and scuttled to the gate. In the end I had to call my friend Janice who got out of the bath, drove round, and set me free – when she'd eventually stopped laughing. Moral of the story: do not try on anything too small when there's nobody else at home.

37 Drink red wine.

Thrilling news from the University of Navarra, who carried out more than 30 studies looking at the effects of drinking alcohol on weight. They concluded that wine drinkers, especially men, were less likely than non-drinkers and people who drank spirits to carry around excess fat.

Then, if that wasn't enough, scientists from Yonsei University in South Korea looked at the super-nutrient resveratrol, which is found in red wine, and found that it may suppress hormones that trigger fat-storing mechanisms. Mice tested showed a significantly lower weight gain than their poor little mates who were not given the resveratrol supplement.

Best of all, the red wine with the highest concentration

of this excellent substance which comes from the grape skins, turns out to be Rioja which is one of my favourites. Win, win, all round.

38 Drink lager.

I don't, because I really don't like the taste, but *Times* columnist Carol Midgley, who is enviably slim, swears by it.

"I truly believe that alcohol calories are not the same as cream cake calories," she tells me. "Lager doesn't make you fat." What she describes as her "dearly-cherished (possibly delusional) theory" goes, as she once wrote in *The Times*, like this:

- Lager is mostly water and passes through you so quickly that you spend most of the evening tripping to the pub toilets, thus burning off more calories than wine drinkers.
- Lager is fizzy and therefore filling, so you feel less compunction to go off and eat, unlike wine drinkers, who seem perpetually obsessed with food.
- The association of lager with beer bellies is a red herring.

She explains the latter thus: "Some men with big stomachs do indeed drink beer, but it is the steak and kidney pie and chips that they tend to buy from the chippy on the way home from the pub that is the culprit. Lager is just the innocent fall guy." She is backed up in this claim by research at University College London and the Institute of Clinical and Experimental Medicine in Prague, which found "no link" between the amount of beer people drink and their stomach size.

Carol goes on to declare that there are fewer calories in a half of lager than in a 175 ml glass of wine (true) and that at least lager makes one a happy drunk whereas "wine makes for weepy ones".

I am not entirely sure about the latter – I always think any sort of alcohol enhances whatever you started with. If you start in jolly celebratory mood you end up dancing on the table; if you have had a hell of a day and are already at the chin-quivering stage, you finish the evening sobbing in a corner.

It also, as we know, blunts the inhibition mechanism. Hence, if one is annoyed by, say, one's partner's irritating ways that have been getting on your nerves all bloody week, one no longer seethes quietly when he says something deliberately galling, but is liable to throw one's handbag at his head. (Or, in one inglorious moment in my own marriage, the fairly large and solid wooden pepper grinder that happened to be close at hand. Don't worry, he ducked.)

Carol also maintains that beer or lager doesn't produce anything like the hangover that wine does. I wouldn't know as I have never drunk either of the former, but this is possible as it is bound to be less dehydrating than wine (with which you should always have a glass of water, and preferably suitable snack) but I'm not sure she was quite right when she concluded one article with "I may be arrested for saying this but a few all-day benders can actually assist weight loss because two bottles of champagne doesn't half kill the appetite."

Hmmm. Not mine it doesn't …

39 Eat crisps.

I like crisps and I work them into my regime in that I have a handful (or two) most nights. Sometimes I chop up a raw chilli and eat that alongside (are you feeling an obsession coming on here?). I must say I do like the upmarket sort (we're back on the crisps now – chillies simply come as little thin ones, or larger fat ones – if you are going to eat them raw I suggest the latter!).

And here Carol Midgley and I again, sadly, part company.

I like the hand-fried kind – Kettle Chips, Waitrose's own version etc. – the kind of crisps that are thicker and crunchier and are simply potato, sunflower oil, and salt (nothing to frighten the horses there). Whereas Carol HATES them (the capitals are hers). "I simply can't be doing with posh crisps," she declares. Adding "Plus, they call themselves 'chips', which is American and that annoys me. Do you think I need to get out more?"

Not at all, love. We can agree to differ on the thickness of our deep-fried potato slice. Any woman who necks back lager, eats any sort of crisps at all, and is still as thin as a pin, is all right with me.

40 Don't drink (at least not all the time).

Yes, I know what the subtitle says – I promised you wine as well as chocolate – but there is no doubt, sad as we may be about this, that alcohol has calories too. And that if you cut back on your booze you will probably lose weight. I say "probably" because I personally find the temptation to eat three chocolate nut cookies in the afternoon, on the basis that I won't be having that Rioja with dinner, almost overwhelming.

But reducing the amount you drink has other benefits as well as its effect on flab-control.

a) There are probably fewer calories in three chocolate nut cookies than there are in half a packet of Kettle Chips, some peanuts, and a cheese straw (with-wine nibbles have a lot to answer for).

b) One definitely looks brighter-eyed, clearer-skinned, and feels more energised in the mornings on mineral water than one does on Pinot Grigio.

c) If you suffer from anxiety and tend to wake up at four in the morning, heart pounding, thinking Oh-my-God-I've-got-so-much-to-do-today (not to mention oh-my-God-what-did-I-do-last-night?) you may find drinking a little less leaves you calmer and more balanced.

On this note, I have been reading *The Sober Revolution* (Accent Press) by Sarah Turner and Lucy Rocca and they do the psychology of being dependent on wine o'clock as the way to de-stress at the end of a tough day, very well. It is worth a read. Even if you don't have a drink "problem" it may speak to you on some level. I have been making a conscious effort to have booze-free days since reading it – which works very well with some of the other strategies outlined in this book, e.g. Going Raw, Intermittent Fasting, or Cutting Out Sugar. If you need an extra incentive, see it as a beauty treatment.

d) You will have more willpower sober, than you can ever hope to harness when three sheets to the wind. Which is why you should:

41 Never drink on an empty stomach.

If you thought your resolve was weakening before, alcohol will see if off altogether. There is a reason why a pre-dinner drink is called an appetiser.

You might be entirely restrained all day but I guarantee that if you have one mouthful of wine when you're even slightly peckish, you'll be in that fridge like a tramp on a kipper.

Have your protein snacks first, or only drink with a meal. (This is the moment to do as I say, not as I rarely do.) And as an added thought to conjure with, you may find you take in fewer calories overall this way.

I have a theory that we sometimes think we want a drink when actually we are hungry. Wine o'clock comes and we think we are gagging for a large glass of dry white when in fact we probably need food. So we either eat things *with* the wine while we're making dinner (if we are like me) or we show due control and restraint on the food front (if we are not) but knock back even more wine, so by the time dinner does come, we are absolutely bloody ravenous and eat everything in sight.

If you are a pre-dinner drinker, just try this as an experiment. It will feel a bit strange, but instead of wine or a gin and tonic, try a nice cup of tea and a chocolate biscuit – or a black coffee and some cheese. Then see if you still want the alcohol with the same fervour.

Or, if you really do not fancy doing that, simply don't drink any alcohol at all until you are halfway through your evening meal. I bet you subsequently drink (and eat) less than you usually do. (Feel free to berate me if you don't!)

42 Eat breakfast, lunch, and dinner.

I have heard very slim people attribute their slender frames to the fact that they never eat between meals and I certainly know a couple of women who live by this rule and both are tiny. I would say it works for me too but because of my somewhat chaotic lifestyle and inability to stick to routine for long, I do not practise it on a daily basis.

The idea is that you eat your three meals a day but you *only* eat then. You never, ever, have anything in between except no-calorie drinks like water or tea or coffee (if you are one of those strange people that likes milk in the latter, I suppose it's OK to have a splash, but no great buckets of coke or double scoop ice-cream milkshakes every hour).

Then you eat breakfast, lunch, and dinner and nothing else. It works especially well if you follow the old adage of eating breakfast like a king, lunch like a prince, and dine like a pauper, or, as I prefer to think of it: Have a fat girl's breakfast, a slim boy's lunch, and eat as little as possible without actually falling in a heap in the evening. (Or certainly some nice lean protein and veg rather than a dustbin-lid-sized stuffed crust with burger topping, double fries, and an entire trifle.)

I believe in this as a principle because of the number of times I have been away at a conference, or been teaching on a writing holiday, or even been staying with gastronomically-minded friends who produce three delicious spreads a day, and found that despite my fears and the fact that I've eaten three full meals a day – sometimes of two or three courses each, I haven't put on any weight. Why? Because there's been no time or inclination to eat anything else apart from at the appointed times and because actually if you add up the calories of three well-balanced meals against those ingested on a day spent picking at bits and pieces, you are probably actually eating fewer! (Even if in the following case, you eat more as the day goes on.)

Compare and contrast:
Breakfast: Fried egg, rasher of bacon, a sausage, grilled tomatoes, a slice of toast and butter;
(Or a bowl of fruit, a yoghurt, a croissant and butter.)
Approx. 500 calories
Lunch: Poached salmon with a blob of mayonnaise and salad, cheese and biscuits. Approx. 600 calories.
Dinner: Soup and bread roll with butter, chicken breast in a cream and mushroom sauce (beloved of all conference caterers), new potatoes, green veg, and carrots.
Apple tart and cream. Coffee with a chocolate mint. Approx. 900 calories.

Still, even on those three meals, you've had no more than 2000 in total (I have rounded up rather than down) which if you you've been walking about, working hard, had the adrenalin flowing, and have that walk before bed, should leave you unscathed tomorrow.

On the other hand imagine a day where you don't really have a "meal" at all:

Nothing but coffee when you get up.

Followed by a muffin when you get to work and another coffee and a KitKat at 11 am. A cheese roll and a bag of crisps when you shoot out at lunchtime – eaten walking back to the office – a couple of biscuits at your desk with a cup of tea at four o'clock, a packet of peanuts in the pub at 6pm when you have a G & T before you go straight onto a work-related reception where you have three glasses of wine, two mini Yorkshire puddings with beef and horseradish, three tiny pastry tart things, and one of those little cones of fish and chips.

As you haven't had dinner you take one of the miniature cupcakes on the way out and have a Twix on the bus on the way home.

It's past 10 p.m. when you get in and you need to get up early tomorrow. By the time you've fed the cat and had a domestic because you haven't been home to eat with your partner since last Wednesday, it's time to hit the sack, you're knackered but you still feel hungry, because as you say – quite accurately – you haven't had a moment to sit down and eat all bloody day! So you feel justified in having some cheese and biscuits or a piece of buttered toast. "I've hardly eaten a thing," you say, as you grab a couple of chocolates from the box or eat a cold sausage from the fridge.

In fact you've consumed upwards of 2,200 calories with the only fruit being the blueberry pieces in your muffin and not a vegetable in sight, and now you're going to lie down and let it all turn to flab. Which is why there are lots of slim people who laugh in an irksome manner and say they eat "all the time", and plenty of podgy ones who are genuinely bewildered about why they are several stone overweight when they really don't eat much, honest.

All are telling the truth as they see it.

43 Eat breakfast.

Sometimes we simply can't manage three balanced meals a day but if you can, try to eat breakfast. If you spread the food from our conference or holiday day the other way round and really go for it at breakfast and have fruit and yoghurt *plus* eggs, sausage, bacon, hash brown, mushrooms, and toast for breakfast, followed by one of those dinky little pastries because they are so hard to resist ... and just the salmon and salad for lunch (with possibly the cheese but lose the biscuits), and in the evening, simply have the chicken and the green veg and go straight to coffee, you will have had the same number of calories but will perhaps even lose a few ounces because research has shown that eating less as the day goes on results in greater weight loss than spreading your intake evenly.

A study published by The Obesity Society cited an experiment carried out by researchers at Tel Aviv University in which two groups of overweight women were both put on a diet of 1400 calories a day. All lost weight (as well they might!) but the group eating 700 calories for breakfast, 500 calories for lunch, and only 200 calories for dinner lost far more than those doing that in reverse (i.e. a 200 kcal breakfast, 500 kcal lunch and 700 kcal dinner).

In addition, the big breakfast group were found to have lower levels of insulin, glucose, and fat in their blood (all good news on the health front) and, most significantly, lower levels of the hormone Grehlin, which, you may recall, is the little devil that increases our appetite.

This meant that the women on the breakfasts felt more satisfied for the rest of the day. Researchers concluded from this, therefore, (if I may so précis) that the body may follow certain rhythms that affect the release of hormones and the way the body processes food, and that if it were going to react so favourably to being fed more earlier in the day, then the fat girl's breakfast could possibly be the way to go. I certainly find that I can eat pretty much anything if I do it early enough in the day. It is the late night feasts before immediately hitting the sack that will layer on the lard.

44 Eat eggs for breakfast.

Studies have shown that if you eat eggs for breakfast you will consume, on average, 400 calories less during the rest of the day than you will if you have a carbohydrate-only based start to the morning. Research carried out over eight years by Dietician Dr Carrie Ruxton showed that those eating eggs, as opposed to cereal, felt fuller for longer and therefore ate less later on. This is presumably because eggs are high in protein, which stops you feeling hungry – and also, apparently, contain quite a specific sort of protein at that, which works well on feelings of satiety. More research is required but eggs may possibly affect some appetite-related gut hormones aiding feelings of fullness, and certainly contain Vitamin D which regulates the amount of calcium and phosphate in the body and promotes strong bones and teeth.

Eggs are also excellent as a hangover remedy and, together with cress and mayonnaise, make the best sort of sandwich.

My quick egg breakfast – and yes it really is filling!

Put a small slosh of chilli oil (you can buy this ready-made or make it yourself by infusing dried chillies in olive oil) or plain olive oil if chilli is a step too far first thing, in a bowl, and add a beaten egg (or two if you are extra hungry). Add some chopped chives or basil leaves or dried chillies if fancied, with a little pile of chopped ham (ditch this if you are a veggie obviously) and some grated cheese. Add black pepper. Stir in a large spoonful of fromage frais. Pop in the microwave on full power for one minute. What you get is a sort of sloppy omelette. If you don't want it sloppy, omit the fromage frais. Either way, it is quick, it tastes good, and you won't want to eat again for ages. Though sometimes I follow it with a couple of squares of dark chocolate. (Just to be on the safe side.)

Alternative slow egg breakfast.

Or you could scramble them. Without wishing to brag, scrambled eggs is one of my specialities. But the secret is to do them S L O W L Y so maybe this is one for the weekends. If you have a large pile of egg lavishly made with milk and butter and black pepper on a slice or two of robust brown bread (the wheat 'n' rye quarter from Waitrose makes brilliant crunchy toast) as a mid-morning brunch, it will keep you going till at least four. (If you do start getting peckish at three, you can just wait a bit!) You'll end up eating less than if you had a more moderate breakfast and then ate lunch. Trust me.

45 Eat eggs generally.

Eggs used to get a bad press (I always ignored it) for their cholesterol content, with advice from on high being to only eat three a week or some such, which always seemed a shame.

There is nothing more versatile than the humble egg and they are the most brilliant weight-control aid as they are filling, nutritious, easy to cook, and you can do so many things with them.

So good news: apparently we can eat them again. It turns out eggs don't have as much cholesterol in them as they used to – something to do with what the hens are fed on these days – and as well as plenty of vitamin D, contain selenium, an important trace mineral, which the most recent research suggests may protect us against some cancers.

So why not have a lovely omelette – let yourself go with what you put in it – with salad, or lower a poached egg into your soup. Have scrambled eggs with smoked salmon, strips of ham, prawns or asparagus, make a filling tortilla or serve up a cheese soufflé – dead easy to make but looks impressive – as long as you don't open the oven door too soon! (Recipe at the back). Or make that fabulous egg mayonnaise sandwich. This was my contribution to the Help for Heroes Cookbook[4] – a publication I can thoroughly recommend. It may not immediately appear to be helping you lose weight – there are some seriously yummy recipes in there – but remember, with the Fight the Flab method, it

Footnote 4 A great collection of recipes from all sorts of people you've heard of (plus me) offered to their heroes (mine raised some eyebrows at the time!) A fab book and such a good cause.

is all about give and take. You can fill your boots today and balance it all out tomorrow – so make a glorious sandwich, have some crisps with it, and a glass of chilled white wine (I like a white burgundy like Macon Blanc Villages) but eat it early in the day, walk before bed, or make that your dinner after a tiny lunch.

46 Cut your salt.

Yes I know one needs salt on an egg but apparently we could all cut down a bit (I'm quite sure I could!). Salt itself contains no calories but it does encourage the body to retain water which in turn will make you *feel* fatter and weigh more. Which you may find dispiriting and since controlling your weight is as much about your state of mind (remember "Thinking Thin") as the food you eat, we don't want that. Too much of the salty stuff isn't great for your blood pressure either so it's worth keeping an eye on how much you're taking in – particularly if you're eating a lot pre-packaged/processed foods which are often the main culprits.

47 Eat to your own rhythm.

This isn't always possible I know – work, life, family can get in the way – but if you get the chance to experiment with eating when *you* want to, rather than when circumstances and social convention dictates, it is worth trying. We are talking listening to your body again – and ignoring the clock and eating when you really feel hungry – and also eating what you want to eat. Because I can't help feeling that a lot of weight is sometimes piled on by living under a traditional (often bloke-controlled) regime where one eats three meals a day at the same set times, because that's what one's (his in particular) mother always did! It may be you find if you tune into your genuine hunger signals that you eat somewhat less.

For example, I'm never hungry as soon as I wake up, I need to have been up and wandering about for quite a while before I'm ready to eat. So, on a day working at home, and left to my own devices, I like to eat a sort of brunch – probably between 10 and 11 a.m. That means I don't need much, if any, lunch but I do get hungry at about 4 p.m. And, if I think I'm going to be having dinner later, I'll have something small to keep me going (quite often chocolaty or biscuity) but if I were home alone, and not going out that evening, then I might eat a proper meal and that would be it – maybe a glass of wine in the evening …

Not every day is the same of course. I get up at different times and my level of hunger varies, but as a general rule on the days I'm at home, with no social demands, I no longer eat breakfast *and* lunch, but one or the other, or the brunch I mentioned. I was fatter in the days when I always ate lunch with my husband, who also worked mostly from home and is the sort who eats at 8.50 a.m., 1.10 p.m. and 7 p.m., and begins to twitch if the schedule slips. But I realised after a while it was simply a habit and one I discovered I could do without.

I once lost weight without trying at all because I was compèring a show at the local theatre. What with rehearsals and then and then the three-night run, I couldn't eat dinner at the usual time for over a week, but since I didn't want to skip it altogether/eat very late because I needed the sustenance for energy/that is a sure route to weight gain, I ate properly at around four in the afternoon and then when I got home at 11 p.m. ish, I unwound with a glass of red wine and a small handful of roasted peanuts.

I expect the adrenalin from performing helped, but I wasn't hungry and the weight came off steadily all week, because I was having my main meal early, doing exercise after that, and only eating protein in the evening. If you are able to spend a few days – or preferably weeks – eating exactly when you want to, and only then, it is interesting to see how it affects the scales.

48 Eat little and often.

This rhythm might suit you better – remember this book is all about finding out what sings to *you* – and there is an argument for doing it anyway. Because the more often you eat the more often you will raise your metabolism. People who struggle with their weight often really don't appear to eat much – I have big friends who do not seem to eat any more – or indeed less – than I do but if you study their eating patterns they often go all day on nothing but a black coffee and then go a bit mad in the evening. Which, a bit like binge drinking, is not a particularly great idea.

But see how you get on – if you are going to count calories it is probably better to spread your allowance out over the course of the day, just to stop you ending up totally famished and liable to say "to hell with it, I don't care about having a big bum anyway." Which can happen all too often on any diet.

But if your own rhythm is graze all day, and have three

meals, plus snacks at bizarre times – perhaps you are one of these people who say they can't possibly sleep unless they have just filled their stomach with cornflakes or cheesecake – and you still want to have the full range of foodstuffs at your disposal, with wine and chocolate of course, then the only foolproof way to definitely control your weight is the tried and tested:

49 Count the calories.

This, of course, is the only way to be able to eat all foodstuffs all the time. You develop a scientific knowledge of the calorific value of everything you are likely to want to consume and keep a running total in your head. Or, nowadays, naturally, there are computer programmes, websites, apps, and all sorts to help you, although even these cannot solve the knotty problem of what to do when you were heavy-handed with the bacon at breakfast, you were unexpectedly invited out to lunch, have already consumed 1654 calories when your upper limit was 1500, it's only 3 p.m., and you're starving. Calorie counting is totally foolproof and works like a dream as long as **you stick to your allowances**.

To do this successfully you have to approach the calorie controlled diet with military precision, a will of iron, and a degree in forward-planning. This is not to say it cannot be done.

Morgen (yes it is spelled with an "e") Bailey, the wonderful woman who builds my blogs and calmly sorts out my technical issues when I am flapping, has recently written **All it Takes is Willpower and Maths – How I Lost 2lbs A Week.**

I only got my first whiff of this when she walked into a restaurant to meet me after I'd not seen her for a while and there was something about her I couldn't quite put my finger on. "You look glam, love," I said, scanning hair, clothes, inner glow. "I've lost two stone," she said, unfazed when I grabbed my notebook, Flab-Fighting antennae twitching.

"I've been inspired by your tips," she said, (one of the blogs she built was 100waystofighttheflab.com) "and I'm only eating when I'm hungry." But further interrogation revealed that actually, she'd also been calorie counting.

Here's her story (I was going to remove the nice bits about me but then my ego thought better of it):

"Between January 1999 and June 2013, I had let five stones (70lbs, 32kg) creep on to my body. I loved, and still love, food. And we need to eat, don't we? The trouble is I was eating all the wrong things and too many of them. I knew what I was doing. No one loses weight stuffing their mouths with chocolate bars and crisps. A special man in my life made me realise that I wasn't happy being single but before I could feel good with someone else, I had to feel good about myself. I'd been on various diets before, official and unofficial. I'd weighed out food, cut out food, but those that had worked (not many did), hadn't worked for long, so I needed a new approach. And my own way of doing it. I was also not only inspired by the tips on Jane's *100 Ways* blog and e-book, but by Jane herself; her bubbly personality, her seemingly unending enthusiasm. I'd had that once. And I wanted it back.

So I went back to basics. I didn't cut out any food but made sure I knew the calorie content of what I was eating.

Women are recommended to have no more than 2,000 calories a day, men 2,500 a day, and surprisingly it goes quite a long way. Sure, I get weeks when I lose momentum but I only have to look in the mirror (I've sold my now-outsized clothes!) and remind myself why it's worth it."

Morgen is still losing weight and looking fab. Here are some before and after photos just so you can see I haven't made her up:

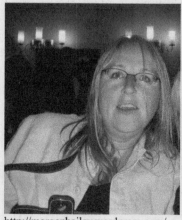 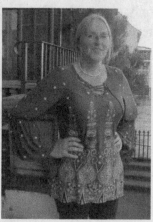

http://morgenbailey.wordpress.com/

But if you don't have Morgen's discipline and ability in mental arithmetic, you could always embrace my very own technique and uniquely-original plan and go on:

50 The shelf diet.

This stroke of genius was created by the heroine, Cari, of my very first novel, *Raising the Roof*, published in paperback by Transworld in 2001 and still available on Kindle etc. (in case, instead of eating so much, you want to take pity on a poor impoverished author and go buy a copy).

I am still shocked that, considering its sheer brilliance, I am the only person to have thought of it (and hurt that as yet, nobody has fallen over themselves to commission me to write an entire ten-volume series on the subject or – recognising that I am sitting, no longer on a bad case of Writer's Bottom, but on a diet breakthrough, given me my own TV series).

It works like this:

You take one shelf of your fridge and each day put on it exactly one thousand calories worth of food – no more, no less. Then you eat it.

There are other rules of course. Like you can't eat anything else that's **not** on the fridge shelf.

Its wonderful simplicity lies in the fact that it's all planned beforehand. No wandering around the kitchen wondering what you dare eat. Temptation is removed, all the calculation is done before you start and you never feel deprived because there's always all that food waiting for you.

When you stock your shelf you make sure it is beautifully balanced with a combination of fats and fibre, sweet and savoury, so you can open the fridge door and say: Hey! What shall I have now? An apple or a Mars bar? And know you still have three boiled eggs, four bits of Ryvita, and a tin of sardines in brine to choose from until bedtime!

To this end, I recommend in fact preparing the whole week in advance – allowing one the flexibility of popping a bottle of chilled white in the door – and filling the fridge with seven or ten thousand calories (this remarkable system allows for a choice of fast-tracking or slower weight loss) worth of food on which you live exclusively for the next seven days. This may need to be adjusted if you have plans to eat out, have the sort of friends likely to arrive unannounced clutching a curry, or live with a bloke who cannot grasp which shelf of the fridge he's got to keep his mucky hands off.

Once word gets around – and I'm relying on you here, fame has been a long time coming – I am expecting to be mobbed by an eager public demanding I write the entire full-length Shelf Plan with colour photographs, a different shelf combination for every day, and/or full fridge option for every week of the year.

And in time, when the world is losing weight and falling gratefully at my feet, there may well be a supermarket franchise with shrink-wrapped plastic trays containing a day or week's choices, pre-calorie-counted and all ready to carry home and place directly on the fridge shelf with no need to spend valuable time preparing it yourself. (An excellent alternative for those unfortunate enough to have gluttonous husbands and ghastly children filling the fridge with their own dubious food.)

In the meantime, once again we have a diet where anything goes. Fancy a jam doughnut? Pop it on the shelf. A sausage sandwich your thing? Have it!

For you are in control of what's on offer tomorrow. As long as you remember these golden rules –

Prepare your shelf the night before. (Preferably when you're not starving) so it's all ready for breakfast and there's no risk of getting overcome with malnutrition first thing and gulping down four slices of toast and a fried egg sandwich you hadn't bargained for.

Make the shelf look full. If all it's holding is a large bag of crisps and a chocolate biscuit, anyone can see you're going to be tempted to ram these down for elevenses and have a very sad evening. This is where the full-week plan comes into its own.

Then you can stick in the in the crisps *and* biscuit but fill up the spaces with 6032 calories worth of worthier items.

Carrots and tomatoes are good, as are huge bags of salad. Half a dozen eggs looks substantial and at only 480 calories leaves thousands of spare calories for Cadbury's chocolate fingers[5] (one of Cari's favourites).

These are especially good shelf components being under 30 calories each and fourteen – two a day – looks such a wickedly indulgent pile of chocolate delight that you'll soon forget you're on a diet at all. (Imagine the sheer joy of a scheme where you can eat fourteen biscuits and still have 6,482 calories worth of food to devour and end up looking stunning.)

Don't have friends round. They will mess things up by attempting to eat the crisps with you and sharing your wine. (Then what will you drink tomorrow?)

Footnote 5 You would think, wouldn't you that after all these name checks for Cadbury's Chocolate Fingers, Burton's Foods Ltd who make them would have the decency to send me down a lorry-load. I'm still waiting …

Don't go out. And if you do, don't eat anything. (Unless you've deducted accordingly from fridge components.)

Be healthy. If all you've got in the fridge is cake, take a vitamin pill.

If it goes wrong, which it sometimes does – warning signs: you have half a lettuce and three radishes to last four days – don't despair! Remember nobody's perfect. Eat everything in the fridge, have a large glass of wine, and start again tomorrow.

NB please send your grateful testimonials to shelf@janewenham-jones.com. 'Before' and 'After' pictures welcome.

51 Plan ahead.

Even if you don't want to follow my excellent diet scheme above (shame on you), a little pre-planning can go a long way. It is much easier to eat moderately and healthily if all the components are close at hand.

An hour spent making your own "salad bar" for example – chopping up onions and peppers, grating carrot, shredding cabbage, washing cherry tomatoes, and storing it in containers in the fridge – will give you no excuse not to pile your plate high with crunchy goodness for the next three nights instead of just heating up another pizza and having it with oven chips.

If you decide on your menus for the week ahead, shop for those meals in advance – sticking to that list of ingredients and nothing else – and do any preparation you can beforehand, e.g. making a pasta sauce or casserole and putting in the freezer, you will be far more likely to keep to your intentions.

NB It goes without saying that it is best not to do the above shop when you're hungry. Not unless you want to come home with enough food to last till Christmas.

52 Keep magazines in the fridge.

This is a celebrity tip, included by kind permission of novelist Katie Fforde. Katie's logic goes like this. A lot of the time we eat because we're bored. If you find reading material in the fridge you can peruse that instead. I might also add that it is useful to keep nail varnish in there too. It stops it going lumpy. And if you're that bored, you can paint your nails when the magazine's finished.

53 Keep busy.

Better still, don't get bored in the first place. If you're starting to feel peckish, throw yourself into the next task, project, or episode of *Downton Abbey* and attempt to get so deeply involved that the gnawing sensation in your middle becomes very much of a secondary consideration.

Attack each task with vigour and enthusiasm as if it were the most important thing you had to do ever, and tell yourself you can eat when it's done. It's all about mindset.

If you were right in the middle of auditioning for a part in a movie with your favourite star/meeting the Queen/phoning the lottery helpline with the winning six numbers or playing in goal for Chelsea, you wouldn't be thinking about where your next sandwich was coming from, would you?

54 Do that food combining lark.

You know that little number made famous by the Hay Diet whereby you can't eat protein and starch at the same meal? The idea is that by eating either one or the other the stomach digests it all more efficiently or some such. It does work – I've tried it – and devotees of the regime tend to have a definite glow (this could be more smug virtue at having lost weight while the rest of us still have several chins) but there is a reason why.

Once again, you can't help but eat less. Suddenly Fish *and* Chips is a no-no, as is sausage and mash, toad-in-the-hole, any sandwich unless it just contains lettuce, cheese on toast, shepherd's pie – you get the picture. It is the variety – the combinations of textures and flavours that keeps us eating (as the fast food industry has so successfully proved with its blending of fat, salt, and sugar) and once you have to have half a favourite meal in isolation you won't eat so much. Give it a try though by all means. See if it irritates you as much as it did me.

55 Whiten your teeth.

Bright gnashers are always attractive and one of those kits where you have put the bleaching gel in the rubber dental moulds and clamp them over your teeth for hours on end are relatively inexpensive and effective. They also make it totally impossible to eat.

56 Find your Achilles Heel.

When it comes to eating to the point of spare rolls and love handles, we all have a weakness that is largely responsible.

For some it is chocolate, for others it might be beer or ice-cream. Personally, I can do perfectly well without biscuits or cakes (even if I am rather partial to a chocolate finger) but have a ridiculous weakness for crisps. Not to mention peanuts, small savoury biscuits, cheese straws – basically anything highly calorific that is salty and goes well with wine!

It started when I gave up smoking over two decades ago and was looking for a replacement for the always-have-one-with-a-drink fag. Now when six o'clock comes and I hit the kitchen in search of corkscrew or gin bottle I am rooting around for a little bowl of something to eat too. This is bad on all sorts of levels.

It means I am using up about a quarter of my daily calorie allowance (if I happened to be counting calories which I'm usually not) on something that is not particularly nutritious or filling and just makes me want more of it. If I took the plunge and stopped both wine and crisps for a week I'm sure I'd shed weight without making another single change to my lifestyle.

But suppose that feels a bit drastic? (It is 5.55 p.m. now and it does!). The trick is to find a replacement. Identify your area of downfall and line up a less calorific/lower fat/more filling/healthier alternative and get that down your gullet instead.

I have discovered the Food Doctor range of Corn & Soya Crisp Thins in what they describe as "exciting natural

107

contemporary flavours" (so far I've tried the Sweet Chilli and Mild Korma). These are made from 50% corn and 50% soya and are "popped" rather than baked or fried. High in both protein and fibre. Sounds dull – tastes surprisingly good. Perfectly acceptable, anyway, as a pre-dinner with-wine nibble and only 95 calories a bag. So you can save on the calories or eat twice as many!

OR – Katie Fforde gave me this great tip too: which is to take Ryvita, and sprinkle it with finely grated cheese (I add chopped chilli but then I would, wouldn't I!) and put them in the microwave for 30 seconds.

Depending on the variety (we both like the seedy ones), and how generous you are with the cheese, you can eat three of these and still be batting around 250 calories.

As Katie says: "They end up very crunchy and tasty and a bit filling. A good 'crisp' substitute, I think." I think so too.

So – If your weak spot is say – the contents of a box of chocolates at that low blood sugar hour of the late afternoon (I have been there too) then you might want to prepare, say, a bowl of strawberries instead or some low-sugar sweet you can suck.

If you have a tendency to hit the cheese and biscuits at 9 p.m. then be ready with the carrot sticks and zero-fat yoghurt dip (yes I too can see that might not hit quite the same spot but you get the idea). If you're basically huge because you can't resist the bedtime Arctic Roll, sausage sandwich, and stuffed crust pizza with your cocoa I'm not quite sure what to suggest. Could you get your jaw wired?

57 Prepare little protein snacks.

The important thing, whether you're actively trying to lose weight or simply maintain your current size and not descend into dispiriting grossness before next Tuesday's work's do, is to never let yourself get too hungry.

When you're really hungry, resolve will go out of the window. You'll tell yourself you don't actually give a damn if your backside won't fit through the door, and anyway you can start again next week.

All that matters at that moment of gnawing starvation is that you get that double club sandwich down your neck and get it down fast. This is where a little pre-empting comes into its own.

Make sure you have plenty of healthy, filling, tasty little snacks within easy access. E.g. Quorn cocktail sausages – (you may of course like the full pig variety but I live in fear of grisly bits in the "real" sausage) cubes of cheese, rolls of ham, chopped cooked chicken, nuts, prawns, pots of yoghurt, whatever floats your non-carb boat. I am suggesting protein because this is the most effective food group to bring about a feeling of satiety.

(You over there with the will of iron, feel free to nibble on fruit instead or have a nice glass of hot water.)

If planning isn't your thing, don't forget, as mentioned earlier, that a black coffee and a few squares of that dark chocolate will also work as a stop-gap. Suck the chocolate slowly, do deep breathing and think how proud you'll be when you *can* get that zip up tomorrow.

58 Change the triggers.

As well as identifying what it is you're eating too much of, examine what you're doing while you're eating it. If, for example, you tend to eat all sorts of bits and pieces while you are in the kitchen, mixing and stirring, can you break the habit by choosing things that cook themselves for a while?

I'm thinking of the sort of one-pot dishes, where you stick it all in, bung it in the oven, and go and sit in another room, out of the way, while it turns itself into dinner. A slow cooker can be great here. Do all the chopping and preparation straight after breakfast when you aren't hungry and then leave it to do its stuff for the next eight hours or so. Better still get someone else in the family to cook.

If you always snack when you watch TV can you whiten your teeth then? Or put on such a tight face mask you can't move your jaw? If you snack at your desk, sit on an exercise ball so you're too busy trying not to fall off.

And if you always hit the sweets when you drive the car anywhere, sing to yourself instead. Or practise your French, learn Mandarin Chinese via the in-motor music system, or recite poetry. Anything that can't be done with a gob full of toffee.

59 Practise your own aversion therapy.

When you need to cut back, picture something revolting. A horribly squashed sandwich or the sensation of chewing on a piece of gristle (I am so suggestible I am gagging as I type but you may be made of sterner stuff and need a viler image). My most successful source of aversion came in the form of a friend's child who took in food in such a thoroughly disgusting manner I used to retch watching and could barely eat at all. His mother thought I sat near him because he was lovely.

60 Eat soup.

If you need to shift some weight fairly quickly and don't want to be starving yourself for hours on end then soup can be your salvation. I am not talking about the famous fad: the Cabbage Soup Diet, which involves you eating nothing but soup (and a fairly dull, bland, soup at that) for a week and being sent doo-lally by the monotony of it all (I will reproduce it below just in case you adore brassicas, think you are tough enough, and fancy giving it a whirl) but the consumption of soup generally as a meal replacement, nutritious snack, hunger-diminisher and all-round comfort.

Soup, especially a delicious home-made concoction – though these days some of the more upmarket supermarket offerings are pretty good too – is a great weapon in the fight against flab.

If you are doing low-carb, then have a big bowl of it with some grated cheese on top or even a swirl of cream or aioli – home-made fish soup is especially luxurious like this. If counting the calories it is easy to make a great steaming cauldron of veg-based broth where a couple of whizzed-up potatoes will add body and a silky texture, without breaking the kcal bank. If you are "fasting" you can sip several mugfuls throughout the day for your 500 calories. And if you are wanting to do low-fat then you can make soup without any at all. If you add some chilli you'll be boosting your metabolism and raising your spirits at the same time – the capsaicin, the natural chemical that gives chillies their heat –

is also known to give one an endorphin rush. (Probably why it's easy to get nigh-on addicted to the blighters.)

I've added some soup recipes at the back but there are a zillion available in cookery books and on the internet. Experiment and find the ones that light *your* fire ...

61 Eat cabbage soup ...

Just for your info and in case you want to try it, here are the details of the traditional cabbage soup diet, the origins of which I haven't quite been able to track down. Proponents claim that one can lose up to ten pounds in a week – I'm not sure this is good for you – while others say this loss is only water, and the weight will soon pile back on again. I can't say the plan is grabbing me by the throat as an option but if you are desperate to get your buttons done up by the weekend, do let me know how you get on ...

Method Make vast quantities of Cabbage Soup – recipe at the back.

Follow this plan: (the italics are my own).
Day 1: Eat unlimited cabbage soup and any fruit except bananas. Drink water or sugar-free fruit juice. *(Fruit juice is full of sugar – presume they mean unsweetened by anything extra...)*
Day 2: Eat cabbage soup with additional vegetables. Have one jacket potato with butter for dinner. *(At least there's butter – be grateful for small mercies, etc.)* Eat no fruit at all.
Day 3: Eat unlimited cabbage soup plus fruit and vegetables of your choice (excluding potatoes and bananas). *(Any butter or cheese on the vegetables perchance? Seems not ...)*
Day 4: Eat unlimited cabbage soup plus skimmed milk. You

can also eat up to eight bananas. *(I am feeling no joy at this prospect. Don't like milk, don't much care for bananas. And I imagine by now, the very sight of that soup ...)*

Day 5: Eat unlimited cabbage soup and 565g *(very precise!)* of beef and 6 tomatoes. Drink 6-8 glasses of water today to help flush any excess uric acid from your body. *(I would be hitting the gin, never mind 8 glasses of water)*

Day 6: Eat unlimited cabbage soup and any amount of beef and vegetables (except for potatoes). *(My excitement knows no bounds)*

Day 7: Eat unlimited cabbage soup with a little brown rice, vegetables, and sugar-free fruit juice. *(Beat head repeatedly against kitchen wall to relieve the monotony. Get on scales – and hurl body from bathroom window if not shadow of former self. After a week of that I would expect compensation in the form of miracles ...)*

62 Try eating by fractions.

This is a very simple idea which is designed to ensure you have a balanced diet and keep your weight under control. You take one plate and arrange food on it as per the diagram below.

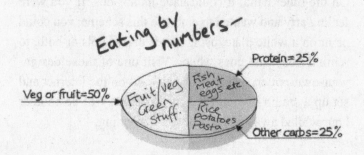

Half the plate should be filled with salad,vegetables, or fruit, a quarter of it with protein: meat, fish, eggs, cheese, quorn etc.; and the remaining quarter with traditional carbs: potatoes, rice, pasta, and so on. I imagine the theory is that if you are sufficiently anal and organised to do this three times a day and not fall on the biscuits in between, you are guaranteed to lose weight/maintain your already sylph-like frame.

I can, however, foresee problems.

- How big is the plate? If it is the size of a washing-up bowl and you fill a third of it with chips three times a day, you could be in trouble.

- How high can you go? Have you seen the way some people pile their plates at the all-you-can-eat buffets? (Have you been to America?) The practised may well fit on five burgers, six sausages, and some bacon into protein, and make a hash brown/Yorkshire pudding tower in the carbs section. And if that's only for breakfast ...

- What do you do about breakfast if you want your scrambled egg *on* toast or something sloppy like porridge? Won't it run into the veg section?

On the other hand, it could have its upsides. If you were feeling arty and wanted to embrace this scheme, you could paint on a white plate, using words or symbols or both, to remind you what goes where. Visit one of those design-your-own-pottery places – or buy a kit on the internet and set up a studio in your kitchen – and that will be another hour whiled away when you won't be eating.

63 Use a plate whatever.

If you make a pledge with yourself that you will never eat anything without putting it on some sort of plate first (even if not a hand-designed one) and then sitting down in front of it, you will be amazed at a) how this slows things down – giving you less time to actually eat and b) how much you usually just casually put straight in your mouth without really thinking about it.

64 Keep good things to munch close at hand.

If you are a nibbler and a picker and found via the above experiment that you are constantly casually popping small snacks into your mouth then make sure you keep good things to munch close at hand. This is also helpful if you are hungry and holding out till the next meal or are trying to wean yourself off your personal downfall. Carrots are useful here (you could also try radishes, celery, or sugar-snap peas depending on your predilections). A medium-sized carrot is likely to come in at under 40 calories and takes a lot of chewing (remember tip number 4?). Chop one into sticks and chomp on it every time you feel inclined to have a chocolate or a bag of crisps. You will get very fed up with carrots, but you will appreciate that praline twirl all the more in due course, and in the meanwhile …

65 Sing!

Singing can burn up to 150 calories per hour, as well as increasing oxygenation in the blood stream, exercising muscles in the upper body and reducing stress levels. It is also quite difficult to eat while you are doing it.

My friend Janie Millman – of whom you will hear more later – and I share a deep-seated conviction that we sing much better after a glass of wine. I confess it was I who, one best-forgotten evening, felt compelled to treat a restaurant in Shepherd Market to a selection of numbers made famous by Elaine Paige but Janie joined in with aplomb. Only one person left and the chaps on the next table were helpful. "It might have been better," said one kindly, when we'd finished, "if you'd both been singing the same tune."

66 Drink lots of water.

Sometimes we think we are hungry when really we are a bit dehydrated and need fluids. There is a theory that drinking a glass of water before each meal will lead to feeling full quicker and therefore eating less, and another that your body needs the water in order to burn fat. Certainly if you are following the high protein approach you should drink lots to prevent putting strain on the kidneys. Water also gives you more energy, flushes out toxins (hot water with a piece of lemon in it is a good detox first thing), and improves your skin no end. Keep a bottle or glass next to you and sip away at it. Or:

67 Drink tea.

Studies on rats have appeared to show that properties in Green Tea boost the levels of the hormone adiponectin in the body (obesity is associated with decreased adiponectin) and some dieters take green tea extract in supplement form. I never have, but I do drink gallons of the liquid stuff. Green tea with lemon, jasmine tea, herbal teas, and also Darjeeling. No milk (ugh) or sugar. This is because I find it easier to drink vast quantities of fluids when they are hot (champagne excepted) and I am probably addicted to caffeine. Yes, green tea has it too, but I believe the wonderful benefits of all those free-radical-busting anti-oxidants it also contains cancels out the negative effects. I am currently rather partial to teapigs which can be ordered on www.teapigs.co.uk – they even have suggestions for teas to drink when you're podgy! If you dig around in the bowels of my blog, you might find a discount code.

68 Drink coffee (or not ...)

The pros and cons of drinking coffee is one of those hotly debated topics giving rise to a whole spectrum of advice that varies according to who's giving it. Many diet books and weight-loss plans instruct you from day one to cut out caffeine, with some dieticians treating it as the drink of the devil.

If you Google coffee and weight loss you will find claims that it helps burn fat and other assertions that the cortisol it produces in the body will do the opposite.

I gave it up for ten years because it was making me blotchy.

And I can't say I have noticed either a positive or negative effect on my weight since I've taken it up again but then I only have on average about a cup or two a day. As I've said, it can be a useful stop-gap between meals (don't forget the chocolate) and it can perk one up when one has hit the late-afternoon low.

Coffee fans will cite its many health benefits from providing antioxidants to protecting one against liver disease to sharpening the performance of the brain.

There are also those who swear by green coffee bean extract as a weight-loss aid – I haven't tried it so have no way of telling you whether it works, but I would certainly be wary of buying any pills, unless I was very sure of what was in them – and there are others who believe in coffee enemas (Eek!).

Summing up: the jury is still out on whether coffee is good for you – you must make your own mind up – but even if it is, I wouldn't want it up my bottom.

69 Do lovely things with vegetables.

Vegetables are low in calories and high in fibre and vitamins. I'm not convinced the world will collapse if you don't eat five a day but there's no doubt that a pile of veg is good for you.

School dinners scarred me for life and I was in my twenties before I learned to embrace broccoli or spinach but I have now learned that if you are creative, vegetables can be interesting, tasty, and filling. So you can eat really big platefuls of them and still lose weight.

I like most vegetables with butter and black pepper. But be adventurous and roast them with garlic, bake them in sauce, stir fry with spices or make a multi-veg curry. Because the vegetables themselves are so low in fat you can add cream or olive oil and still get away with it.

What I really love in the season is eating runner beans as though they were spaghetti – cut into very long thin strips and boiled till just tender, then piled high on a plate tossed with butter, grated cheese, and black pepper.

The best runner beans are the ones you grow yourself and this is surprisingly easy to do even if you only have a tiny back yard, as they can be grown in a tub, up a few canes. Even more excitingly, you can start the beans off in the old fashioned way, in a jar on the windowsill, the beans placed against some wet blotting paper or folded kitchen roll and stage a race.

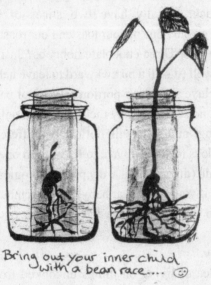

Bring out your inner child with a bean race.... ☺

Star-rating for all-round-interest, healthy-living, and entertainment *****

NB Carnivores, particularly those on a very strict protein diet, may prefer to eschew vegetables (which are, after all, largely carbohydrate) and do lovely things with meat instead.

Personally I can't digest too much dead animal at one sitting and am slightly put off by the way the meat-only brigade have that appalling breath.

Star-rating * OK for those who don't mind if their only friend is their butcher.

70 Eat half.

This is a simple and effective way of losing weight – as long as you keep to it. Just have everything you usually have but half as much. Usually have two slices of bread for breakfast? Pop only one in your toaster. Four roast potatoes? Cut back to two. Three chocolate hobnobs? Just have two of those as well (it's all a bit awkward to leave half a biscuit in the tin). Have a half-size portion of chips or pasta – your vegetables and salad can stay the same – and only fifty per cent pudding, and you will notice the difference quite quickly. It does mean you have to leave food on your plate if eating out (difficult on a deep psychological level, I understand, if you were a war baby) but remember if it ends up stored on your hips, it's wasted anyway.

71 Go raw.

I got the idea of living on things uncooked from Alison Matthews, the power behind www.rawconfidence.com.

I had probably heard about it from celebrities too but I must confess I don't pay particular attention when the super-rich are talking about their weight-loss plans. Mainly because it usually necessitates having your own live-in chef and not leaving the house without a facialist and someone to press your chakra points.

But Alison ... I must say Alison looks fantastic and positively glowing. And this, she told me, was down to embracing a diet that is now 70-80% raw. Having "dabbled in" raw food for years, she decided in 2012 to get down to a serious six-week raw food vegan detox, basically living on vegetables, salad, fruit, nuts, and seeds. "I did the detox for my health," she says "and possibly the bonus of losing a few pounds. Little did I know that it was going to change my life!"

Alison was not particularly unfit but she was carrying, she estimates, about an extra 2 stone. She'd lost weight before but always put it back on. Raw food, "felt different" and by the end of the first week she had already dropped a dress size!

"Raw food is quick and easy to prepare and I found I could taste flavours in food in a way in which I hadn't done before."

In the six weeks, Alison lost a stone and a half and a further half stone came off over the next few months as she continued to eat predominantly raw food.

A year on, the weight has stayed off and as Alison says: "I know, for the first time ever, that it won't go back on. I eat a diet of about 70% raw food and still love it. I also have significantly more energy, great skin for a 50-year-old, and I now pick up a small or size 10 when clothes shopping!"

Inspired by Alison, who has now trained as a Raw Food Teacher and Coach, combining coaching, yoga, and meditation together with raw food nutrition to "help others to be healthier and more energetic", I decided to give it a little go myself.

When she sent me three days of menus to try, for the purpose of sharing the experience with you, I did find it rather daunting – mainly because I'd never heard of some of the ingredients (and I wasn't going to be able to drink). But this was for an initial "detox" so we're basically talking vegan (no animal products at all – no not even eggs or a bit of cheese ☹), no sugar, no alcohol, and nothing heated above 40 ish degrees centigrade (the raw foodies seem to have different views on this – it varies from 104-115 Fahrenheit as a top temperature, depending on who you read).

I wasn't sure how this was going to work so I just told myself *raw*. Because of the strange ingredients and because it involved making things, I enlisted my friend Paula into the trial. She went off shopping, and promised to do a bit of the creative stuff and in the meantime, I fell at the first hurdle, namely breakfast. Here is my report:

Day One: Eat six raspberries (which is the only fruit we have left – must go shopping) and then look around to see what else I can have that is both raw and vegan and I can face at nine in the morning. There is not much. So I cave in and eat two Dr Oetker seeded spelt crispbreads (which are yummy – try them), which obviously have been baked, some shop-bought houmous which clearly contains cooked chick-peas, (apparently it is quite hard to track down raw houmous and when you do, it is a greenish colour), some basil leaves, and four cherry tomatoes. This is quite a nice start to the day, in fact. And I feel very full after. I could have easily had only one crispbread (note to self: take own advice and listen to body). I also drink green tea with lemon which I shouldn't because it contains caffeine (but I am not doing the detox bit, I decide, just the raw).

1 p.m. : Fall at second hurdle. Eat two squares of chocolate. I forgot! I did honestly. It was just there and I absent-mindedly ate it. But I don't think it's the end of the world as it is Green & Blacks and 85% cocoa. The sugars are listed in the nutritional information at 13.8g per 100g. At 30 squares in a 100g bar this means each square will contain one thirtieth of the total sugar which equals 0.46g so two of those, amounting to less than one gram of sugar is hardly worth even admitting to.

NB For your future reference, each square also contains a mere 21 calories so four squares – remember my tip about having this as a hunger-busting snack? – will come to only 84. Way to go!

Still haven't been shopping so have more shop-bought houmous (more cooked chickpeas) and some salad.

Evening: no wine! Drink lots of water and feel bathed in virtue. Capitalise on this by looking pointedly at husband's glass and droning on about the benefits of alcohol-free days and uncooked produce. He eats lamb chops and ignores me.

I consume an avocado and raw vegetable mountain, dressed with olive oil, balsamic vinegar, and the last of the houmous. It is surprisingly filling and I do not need to eat again that evening. (But I possibly have a bit more chocolate).

Day Two: Oh dear, I am due to go to London where I am invited out to dinner. I do feel slightly guilty as I sit in a tapas bar in Pimlico with a glass of red wine in one hand and a large piece of manchego cheese in the other, reading texts from Paula about her detox headache, but it would be rude to start fussing or only eat salad.

Day Three: Text from Paula reads: "Banana, ground flax seed, coconut, and nut milk for breakfast. Quite nice but want Marmite toast and builders' tea …" I do not tell her I am taking full advantage of the hotel's breakfast buffet.

To cheer Paula up, I take a detour via the Wild Food Café in Neales Yard, Covent Garden and get a take-away order of raw "macaroons" which a nice chap called Andy (all the staff have an inner glow) told me were made from coconut, almonds, a sweetener made from dates, and cacao powder, with a goji berry on top. I have to say they were yummy.

Day Four: See Day One with a bit more chocolate.

Day Five: Tried a cabbage salad, some sunflower pâté and a chocolate truffle, made by Paula to Alison's instructions (see Recipes section.) Plus crisps and wine (it was Friday).

What did I learn?

1   There's nothing like being forced to cut out three-quarters of your foodstuffs to appreciate how many things you can usually eat that are healthy and not unduly fattening.

2   Houmous on crispbread with basil leaves and tomatoes is a rather excellent, invigorating breakfast.

124

3   New combinations: who'd have thought raw asparagus dipped in houmous could be so good?

4   After a day of raw veg and no booze, one definitely wakes up more alert. After two days I felt sharper, brighter, and my eyes were somehow clearer. I am going to use it as an occasional health/beauty treatment, if nothing else. Although, since both Paula and I got a couple of spots at one point – clearly the toxins emerging – perhaps not immediately before a big event.

5   One does also start to long for something hot … (Alison recommends a baked sweet potato.)

But Paula, who did the whole thing properly for seven days, is the one to ask. She was so impressed that she is continuing to follow the regime for a couple of days a week: this is what she had to say:

"Doing the raw food diet was much easier than I'd expected. The most difficult thing was having to be a bit more organised to ensure there were available raw foods at hand and I did miss having something hot when it got cold.

The most obvious effect was I had so much more energy. I had been feeling very sluggish in the mornings for the last couple of months and had been going to bed early too. One night I went to bed at my usual 10 o'clock and lay there realising that I just wasn't tired! I also wake up feeling ready to go and generally have bundles of energy. Fantastic!

When I finished the diet and had a bowl of porridge with toast and Marmite I immediately felt my energy sapping away and felt like going back to bed! This has to be psychosomatic surely? (Alison would say not.)

Anyway, yes, I had more energy, my skin was nice and clear (apart from that day when we got the spots …) and there was some weight loss. All good stuff. And amazingly, I never felt hungry. I watched the family coffee cake and chocolate pudding and didn't even fancy any. Which is very strange because whenever I've attempted to diet before I have always craved sweet foods. In fact I made some date/apricot/nut and carob sweets yesterday and they are still in the fridge. I am not even dreaming about them!!

It's hard when you go out for the evening though and I did break it to have a cider or two … (Now she tells me. And there was me feeling guilty about my red wine …)

If you fancy giving "Raw" a go here is a sample three-day plan courtesy of Alison Matthews. For more details visit her website. www.rawconfidence.com.

Raw Confidence

Detox Meal Plan

Week 1

Day	Breakfast	Lunch	Dinner	Treats	Drinks
1	Berry fruit salad	Sunflower pate with oat or rice cakes and salad	Guacamole stuffed mushroom	Tahini energy balls x 1	Filtered water Freshly squeezed juice
2	Flax seeds and coconut bites with fruit	Spinach soup	Sunflower seed burger with salad (optional tomato sauce)	Piece of fruit	Filtered water Freshly squeezed juice
3	Buckwheat and chia seed porridge	Mega salad with oat or rice cakes	Cabbage salad with baked sweet jacket potato	Tahini energy balls x 1	Filtered water Freshly squeezed juice
4	Mango, spinach and avocado smoothie	Sunflower pate gem of a salad	Zucchini pasta with pesto	Piece of fruit	Filtered water Freshly squeezed juice
5	Omega fruit salad	Mega salad with oat or rice cakes	Cabbage salad with baked sweet jacket potato	Tahini energy balls x 1	Filtered water Freshly squeezed juice
6	Flax seeds and coconut bites with fruit	Basil and pepper soup	Nut burger with salad (optional tomato sauce)	Carrot cake	Filtered water Freshly squeezed juice
7	Banana and chocolate porridge	Sushi style wraps	Raw fajitas	Carrot cake	Filtered water Freshly squeezed juice

72 Eat a Tic Tac.

Carry Tic Tacs or any container of diminutive mints and every time you think about eating something, suck one of these instead. It won't be quite the same as a buttered crumpet, but at least nobody will accuse you of having halitosis (though they might well think you're waging a life-long battle against it). Some people recommend using gum in a similar way, but constant chewing, both in myself and others, gets on my nerves, so I don't.

73 Get enough sleep.

It has been fairly well established that there is a link between obesity and a lack of shut-eye. Poor sleep has been shown to increase the levels of certain hormones associated with weight gain and if you are tired, you are far more likely to crave carbohydrates and fatty foods – which is probably why, when I've had too many late nights and early mornings, I get an overwhelming urge to eat chips.

Sleeping for only five hours or less can also lead to a slowing down of the metabolism and a tendency to consume more calories than usual the next day. So aim for seven or eight hours in bed, if you can. It is tricky to eat when you're snoring.

74 Juggle your junk.

If you do crave some nice fatty carbs – and don't we all sometimes – then some "fast" food, I feel, is a better choice than others. For example, you can get a fair old portion of fish and chips from your local chippy for under 1000 calories (I gleaned my information from the National Federation of Fish Friers on www.federationoffishfriers.co.uk) and fish such as cod is, additionally, a useful source of various nutrients such as potassium (which drinking alcohol can deplete), B and D vitamins, and magnesium (helpful in the fight against PMT if you are currently hurling the cutlery about every month).

I also find vegetable spring rolls can hit the I-want-junk spot quite nicely, too. I bought some from Waitrose recently which were only 77 calories each (not much even when I ate three of them), and did obviously contain vegetables (good for one), yet had that pleasing crunchy, salty, deep-fried feel about them, which was reminiscent of a much more diet-busting repast.

Even if you want something much higher in saturated fat, salt, and general wickedness, better to have it and compensate before and after – via lean protein and salad or fruit only, for the meals either side, or skip eating those altogether – than to obsess about it, feel miserable and deprived, and say: sod the whole flab-fighting thing anyway.

75 Get a diet buddy.

In the same way that a gym buddy can work – I used to work out with my friend Heather who was a veritable slave-driver – a pal who also wants to fight the flab can be a great help in keeping going.

If you are very masochistic you could have your own mini weight-watching session and jump on the scales in front of each other weekly.

If you're not, you could simply swap encouraging noises and hot tips, or take turns to prepare carb-free/low-fat/calorie-controlled dinners and deliver them to each other, in the manner of those home-delivery companies that do all the calculations for you.

Or you could just use one of those companies in the first place or buy low-cal meals from the supermarket. I am only here to help.

76 Read yourself thin.

In their book, *The Novel Cure,* Ella Berthoud and Susan Elderkin put the case that all of life's ills can be remedied by reading literature. For obesity they recommend *A Far Cry from Kensington* by Muriel Spark (as it happens I have already given you the most obvious advice it contains in this very work –see tip No. 70) but the authors say there are more subtle pointers at play too. Muriel Spark is a very clever writer so you'll enjoy it anyway. Even if you don't, the value of a good book cannot be underestimated. When we are really gripped by a book we cannot put it down. We cannot stop reading to get dressed, go to work, turn off the light at night. We might not even want to stop to eat …

77 Eat "heavy" foods.

Research has shown that our feelings of fullness are not dependent on calorie values but the volume and weight of the portions. Therefore a bowl of say, porridge, will fill us up for longer than the same number of calories it contains, presented in a croissant. So if you want to fill yourself up on less, have a big salad starter with tomatoes and onions in it, try bulking out your pasta dishes with extra vegetables, and eat an apple and a small flapjack rather than a socking great meringue nest filled with whipped cream …

130

78 Try the MILF diet.

I am more of a MIDSOW (Mother I Don't Want to be Seen
Out With) than a MILF but I was interested in the latest
bible for the aspiring-to-be-sexy older woman. Written by
Jessica Porter, the concisely subtitled: *The MILF Diet. Let
the power of whole foods transform your body mind and
spirit … DELICIOUSLY* is billed as a practical cookbook
for women who want to achieve optimal health and
happiness (I'm sure you chaps can have a go too). It features
a lot of organic whole grains, plant-based proteins, and
"fermented foods" some of which I've never heard of.
Jessica, who claims to have ingested the placenta (dried and
powdered, I believe) after the birth of her son, is another
advocate of cutting out dairy, meat, sugar, caffeine, and
alcohol, says no one wants to cook for her. Can't think why.

79 Wield the iron.

And do the rest of the housework while you're at it. Yes,
life may be short – but there is no doubt that giving the
house a blitz is an excellent work-out. Ironing tones those
arms; dragging the hoover upstairs will help legs and
stomachs. Taking the rubbish out, dusting that top shelf – it
all promotes muscle tone, and fat burning. Not convinced?
I'd rather pay someone else too …

80 Swallow it too.

If you're on a silly diet, make sure you are getting the right
vitamins and minerals. Sometimes cravings are your body's
way of saying what it needs. If you're mainlining chocolate
brazil nuts for example, perhaps you need selenium. If

you're just sucking the chocolate off you might want iron. If you've eaten three doughnuts, four cookies, and an apple pie, and it's only 11 a.m., you want to get a grip before you're the size of Dorset.

81 Get food poisoning.

This is quickest of all. For best effect, go for full-blown salmonella or dysentery so you've got both ends at once and can't even keep fluids down. My most dramatic experience of weight-loss via this method came from a suspect pepperoni pizza in Verona. I was on the bathroom floor for three days and the water bill came to more than the hotel room. I dropped nearly half a stone. Another time, I collapsed on a plane and threw up in the *New York Times*. If Italy or America are a bit too far to go, you can probably pick up a dodgy kebab in the high street.

82 Fall in love.

This works particularly well with someone who doesn't love you back. Then you can spend hours mooning by the phone waiting for him or her not to call, feeling sick with anxiety, and wondering where you're going wrong. Advantages of this plan: you're much too heart-broken to eat. Disadvantages: you're also all red and blotchy and nobody will ever fall in love with you looking like that.

83 Or pretend you have.

Seriously, there is a reason why those in the first throes of passion usually shift a few pounds and that's 'cos he or she has stopped thinking about food all the time and is obsessed with the object of his or her new desire. I also believe that when you are all happy and excited – or adrenalised, as I like to put it (I thought I had invented that word but from the reaction of the spell-check, it seems not) you really do give your metabolism a boost and burn up calories faster.

Or perhaps you just eat less because you are too busy thinking about whether he or she will call or if it would be a bit forward to send a third text in the same half hour and whether tonight's the night you'll wear the sexy shirt or the dress with the buttons all down the front, rather than where your second chocolate biscuit's coming from.

Either way I can recommend trying your best to recreate this mood and mental state – and it doesn't have to involve trying to inject new thrills into your saggy old relationship or leaving him there snoring on the sofa, for the exciting young man who delivers your Amazon parcels.

I find I can induce this state in myself just through small every-day thrills. For example, even when I am only excited about some work- related issue I can actually feel a surge of adrenalin go through me and I start to move faster, twitch about a bit more etc.

So try to fill yourself with enthusiasm for your goings-on whenever possible. Right now, you could get excited about how much weight you're going to lose and how fabulous you will feel when you are slim. And how wonderful it will be if you get into a way of life that keeps you that way and still lets you eat chocolate! Alternatively you could simply:

84 Have lots of great sex.

A good shag can burn up to 400 calories and increases the endorphins in your body leaving you feeling naturally high without resorting to chocolate. Points in favour: you spend all your eating time bonking, and when you do come up for air, you don't want to look unalluring by ramming food down your throat. Points against: if you're single, you might fall in love, decide to get married, and that will be your sex life gone for ever.

Or you could simply forget love and sex and fall in unrequited lust. The novelist Jane Lovering was a runner up in the Fight the Flab competition which was run through 100waystofighttheflab.com in 2013. Her hilarious exercise tip – Bum's Away – goes as follows:

"I recommend placing a large picture of one's object of desire some six feet distant, then practising 'lunging' forward with alternate legs to place a kiss upon said object of desire. Not only does this shape the behind, but it gives necessary practice

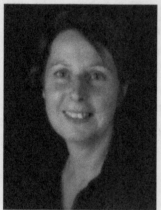

in the 'snog and retreat', which comes in handy should one actually meet the object of one's desire. Aim for ten kisses with each leg. No liability accepted for restraining orders."
Jane Lovering

www.janelovering.co.uk
photo by fresh-photographic.co.uk

134

85 Have a crisis.

(This may follow naturally from above). There are two types of emotional crisis. The one where you are too traumatised to contemplate food and spend a lot of time staring into space feeling tragic, and the sort where only two bottles of wine and half a pound of chocolate, plus chips with houmous will reach the spot. Make sure you develop the right kind. (NB your partner finding out about the great sex probably comes into the first category but it also tends to be very expensive and upsets the children.)

86 Get yourself on TV.

If your other half *has* found out, and there's a brawl brewing, you can always go on *Jeremy Kyle* and share it with the nation. (You might want to consider *Wife Swap* at the same time). Television instantly piles on ten pounds. Once you see the recording, you'll be so horrified you'll never eat again.

NB this was a tip I wrote earlier. My mate Steve, with whom I have just made a TV pilot, has since told me this is a myth. "It may have been true once," he claims, "but not with today's modern cameras and screens." Hmmm. You mean I look like that really?[6]

87 Get pregnant.

I know some women find it a difficult time but I adored being up the duff. What's not to like? You no longer need to think about holding your stomach in and others positively

Footnote 6 see www.wannabeawritertvshow.com and judge for yourself.

135

encourage you to eat. You aren't drinking so you can get the sugar your body is accustomed to by having lots of puddings. If you breastfeed later you can eat even more as someone else is helping to use up the calories. I was thinner afterwards than before I started (this could be because the little blighter didn't sleep through the night till he was about twelve and I was run ragged) although unfortunately I have occasionally made up for it since.

I have never quite recovered from the day in Sharm el Sheikh when an Eygptian waiter looked me up and down, pointed to my protruding stomach and enquired: "You wait baby?"

He nearly got a black eye instead of a tip but there was one small comfort. He thought I was still of child-bearing age.

88 Use a sisal sponge.

I am grateful to the novelist Sarah Duncan for this tip, which she shared with me some years ago. Using a sisal-covered sponge is easier than body brushing but just as excellent in the pursuit of bump-free flesh. Big can be beautiful if it's soft and smooth. Give yourself a good scrub in the shower, with circular, upward movements – always go towards the heart – paying particular attention to potentially flabby areas like bottom and thighs and upper arms with this handy exfoliator and then plonk it on a radiator in winter or hang near a window in summer so it dries quickly and doesn't become grim. You will see and feel the difference, I promise.

89 Don't wear enough clothes.

There is a theory that getting cold activates our "brown" fat (as opposed to the usual blobby yellowish-white stuff) which in turn may burn up calories to try to warm us up again. Research being carried out at the University of Nottingham's Queen's Medical Centre suggests that eventually this brown fat, mostly found around the shoulder blades, strangely, could hold the key to solving weight problems. I am not suggesting you spend your life semi-naked in a walk-in fridge, but when you're freezing your butt off braving snow and gales this winter, you could look on the bright side.

NB An alternative is to wear too many. I've seen these strange folk in the gym, running on the treadmill in three anoraks. Presumably the theory is that you sweat off the pounds. Looks truly horrible. I'd rather strip off. Talking of which:

90 Get painted naked

Or have a good friend photograph you from behind. Both can be a salutary experience. The advantages of being painted, once you have got over feeling thoroughly silly for sitting there in the altogether at 11 a.m. in front of someone you've only just met, is you can always beg your artist to gloss over your ample midriff and double chins. Rose, the wife of Brian Homewood, who painted me, makes no bones about it, "Oh yes," she says airily, "when he paints me, I tell him to make me much blonder and thinner." The camera unfortunately, is less forgiving. I had some "Writer's Bottom" shots taken with the possible thought of using them

137

for the first version of this book. Remember what I said about the importance of motivation? Ye gods …

91 Get some fat friends.
And stay close.

92 Get some thin friends.
And keep your distance.

Big friends may make you feel slender but thin friends will at least shame you. I always eat more around other people who are eating more – if they're on double fries it feels rude not to – and I bet if you think about it, you do too.

Hang out with fat friends, you'll get fatter (but at least you'll enjoy yourself). Go out to lunch with thin friends who toy with their mixed leaves, send the dressing back, and hyperventilate when the bread arrives, and you'll feel too embarrassed to stuff your own face and then go on to have pudding.

93 Trick and treat.
If you find it hard to go too long without your favourite foods then spread them across the week and declare a treat each day. Find out the number of calories each delight contains and then eat round it. If you want a big creamy pudding make the first course a salad. If it's a full roast with crackling, eat soup for the meal before. If you want a deep-fried lunch, have a breakfast of fruit. You might be peckish waiting but the compensation comes when you tuck into all the foods you love and don't need new clothes.

94 Think added incentives.

If you're getting tired of focussing on your fat cells, remind yourself of other benefits too. If you aren't drinking, this will help you look younger. If you are fasting you will also be boosting your general health. If you cut fat you are probably protecting yourself against heart disease. If you give up sugar, your teeth will be in better nick.

And if you read the rest of this book and then tell all your friends about it, I might afford some liposuction.

95 Think Gwyneth.

It means no coffee, alcohol, dairy, eggs, sugar, shellfish, deepwater fish, potatoes, tomatoes, peppers, aubergines, corn, wheat, meat, soy, or anything processed at all, but if you end up looking like Gwyneth Paltrow it could be worth it. And clearly the beautiful actress doesn't eat so strictly ALL the time because her cookbook: *It's all Good: Delicious, Easy Recipes that Will Make You Look Good and Feel Great* contains recipes for Lamb Tagine and Thai-style chicken burgers. But the general focus is on the food she eats when she wants to "lose weight, look good, and feel more energetic". She's living proof that it works, but when I read the list of ingredients I'd have to get, I needed a lie-down.

96 Don't do pills and potions.

Obviously you wouldn't be silly enough to believe the claims of the various ads for miracle cures that promise you will shed a stone in three days, often when you're asleep, and even if you continue to stuff yourself with deep-fried Mars Bars and refuse to exercise.

But just in case you are ever tempted, a small tip. Once, for an article I was writing, my sister and I had an amusing time sending off for various of these "diet pills", the leaflets for which were, at the time, arriving thick and fast on the doormat. We took it seriously, swallowing down horse-sized tablets containing – allegedly – everything from dried grapefruit to seaweed extract, proving they didn't work and then demanding our money back.

All the outfits "guaranteed" refunds if the weight hadn't dropped off, clearly emboldened by the average human's general inertia about returns. And rightly predicting that most people would be so disheartened by finding that – unlike the "before" and "after"s in the leaflet, which we can assume are produced by airbrushing the same fat head onto a thin body – they were still waddling about after a month of swallowing essence of lemon mixed with sawdust, that the last thing they'd feel like was a hike to the post-box.

But on the off-chance they were going to encounter my sister – who has made a career of customer complaints and retrieved us every penny – they'd all cleverly written the return address only on the coupon you sent off with your payment in the first place, or made online instructions for claiming a refund so well buried you needed a degree in archaeology to find it.

So, if you do ever succumb to the urge to spend £49.99 on a few crushed herbs and some talcum powder – and please don't – make sure you know how to send them back first.

97 Don't do "that" diet either.

You know the one I mean don't you? Where you eat nothing at all except a few soupy things and occasional bar things and go for group counselling every week. I'm not entirely sure if you actually have to sit in a circle and say "I'm Jane and I'm a Porker" but the whole emphasis is on breaking old patterns and changing your style of eating for ever. And I strongly suspect that there is a conspiracy afoot to pretend that, during this torture, you are absolutely not hungry at all, ever, because that is what they all do claim. Even if it has been clear to me they are almost ready to bite their own legs off.

I imagine if you are paying quite a hefty fee each week for the whole package that is a fair incentive to stick to it but I can only tell you this. When I once managed to purloin some of the soupy things and the bar things without actually having to go sit in the circle, I tried it for three days.

I sent a text to a friend who was into her fourth month of the regime and had shed about four stone. "I hate this," I texted. "I am fed up, hungry, miserable, bad-tempered, tired, and I have a headache."

She replied with one word: "Welcome."

She was one of six people I know of who followed this diet and all lost shedloads of weight – between three, and an unbelievable seven, stone each. All you need to know is that several years on, every one of them is now back to the exact weight they were when they started.

Stick with me, kids.

98 Avoid five foods.

I expect you, like me, have been bombarded by the ad on the internet that tells you if you just stop eating five foods you will lose weight. You may even have clicked on the button, out of curiosity, and then lost the will to live as the lengthy presentation rumbles on and on – in tune to your stomach – and you're none the wiser. Well, just for you – and you can be forever grateful – I sat all through the whole bloody thing and can now reveal what those five foods that you must never eat again, are. Apparently your excess fat – especially that stubborn "belly fat" – oh yes – will melt away if you can only wean yourself away from:

Concentrated fruit juice (sugar!)

Margarine (trans fats)

Wholewheat bread (carbs)

Processed soy – tofu etc. (can't remember what was wrong with this – think I was nodding off by then)

And genetically-modified corn.

So there you have it. Toss away that tasty lunch of a Soy & GM Corn sandwich, made on wholewheat bread, lovingly spread with best marg., all washed down with a large glass of juice, and your problems will be over for ever.

You're very welcome.

99 Fast Friday, Slim Saturday, and Sinday.

The weekend can be a time of over-indulgence. If you don't want to do the full organised fasting thing, simply make a plan to include treat days and austere times so you can enjoy yourself without piling on the pounds. Keep swapping round the sort of regime you are on to keep up the variety and interest. You might for example, eat raw food all day Friday, do low carbs on Saturday, and then on Sunday have the full cooked breakfast, roast dinner, and a fat pudding. Or just have an apple for lunch on Friday to allow for fish and chips in the evening – focus on the thought of all that crunchy batter when you're wavering over the cream buns at 4 p.m. – decide to mainly live on vegetable soup on Saturday and then Sunday when you're going out for lunch, have the full seven courses, but absolutely no supper.

You could also declare a Munch Monday, Teetotal Tuesday, Waddle Wednesday or a Thin Thursday. The unnecessarily anal may like to make a chart or spreadsheet. It might look like this:

Monday	Big eggs & toast etc. breakfast, low carb rest of day NB take tuna salad to work. Remember drink lots water
Tuesday	Low carb, no sugar, no booze
Wednesday	Eat what like – Gertrude's Hen/Gary's stag night
Thursday	No more than 1800 calories overall (lunch out!)
Friday	Go raw – at least 80%
Saturday	Gary and Gertrude's wedding!!!! (i.e. fill boots)
Sunday	Breakfast like king (will prob need fry-up), lunch like prince, pauper's tiny supper etc. (will prob want hit sack early anyway)

On a week like above you will, if you want to, get to eat cooked breakfasts, a restaurant lunch, yummy party food, and drink wine and champagne, as well as having plenty of fruit and vegetables and I guarantee if you stick to a plan like that you will not put on weight. In fact, if you take that brisk walk before bed and throw in the odd chilli, you will probably lose a bit ...

Here's a blank one, just for you.

Monday	
Tuesday	
Wednesday	
Thursday	
Friday	
Saturday	
Sunday	

100 Be hanged for a sheep.

If you are going to eat something high in calories, fat, sugar, or general loveliness, make it worthwhile. And fabulous.

I cannot be doing with anything involving pretend butter or low-fat cheese or synthetic cream or flavouring. If you want a pudding, have a great big, glorious, chocolatey, cream-covered, alcohol-drenched, celebration of a pudding.

Savour every mouthful and lick the bowl. Better, surely, to do that once a week than hunch over half a stewed pear and fat-free fromage frais daily, feeling dreary.

You can either prepare for it – have something low-cal for the meal before – or compensate later, with brisk walking before bed, and no carbs tomorrow. But enjoy it now. Life is short – and some things are worth enjoying. Which is why if you do go a bit mad, this is not a reason to throw in the towel for evermore. In other words …

DON'T GIVE UP

Just because you fall off the wagon of any given strategy – and we all do! – do not give up on the whole idea of flab-fighting and eat yourself into oblivion.

Let us imagine you are sitting at your desk and feeling stressed and cross and sugar-depleted and tired and grouchy (write what you know, they told me) because you've had a sh*t day and your car's had to go into the garage and your mother-in-law is coming for the weekend and the neighbours kept you awake half the night, and you've still got God-knows-what to get through before you can finish for the evening, and you think: *I will go and make a coffee – caffeine will perk me up – and while I am about it I will have one of those Double-Delight-indulge-why-don't-you, hand-baked, Chocolate-Dipped Cookies that Brenda brought into work and told me to help myself to, because they have nuts in them and the nuts are actually brazil nuts which are high in selenium which is good for stress*, and while you are there at Brenda's biscuit tin, you actually eat four of these large cookies because the sugar depletion bit was more savage than you'd first realised and they were, frankly, absolutely delectable and you could barely stop yourself eating five. So now you are back at your desk washed over with self-loathing thinking: *oh my God that*

*was 600 calories, on top of the toast and peanut butter I had
for breakfast and the pie for lunch and the biscuit that came
with my cappuccino and it's not even 5 p.m. and there's still
dinner to come tonight – loads of it if the mother-in-law's
going to be there, troughing for England – and I'll need a
stiff drink too – ditto …*

Oh well, you think on, *it's too late now – I may as well
eat everything in sight and start again on Monday …*

NO! Stop there. It's that sort of thinking that leads
straight to weight gain. So you do not head back to the
biscuit tin and have three more chocolate chip delights, or
prepare yourself to eat double suet pudding this evening,
you look at it thus.

Even if you have had breakfast, a high-fat lunch, biscuits
and snacks, if you stop right now you probably haven't
exceeded an acceptable calorie intake for a whole day.

Yes, you will be expected to eat dinner when you get home
or your partner will have a face on, but you can just have the
protein and veg or have only a very small portion of
everything. If you are charming to the old dragon and helpful
in the kitchen, your partner will be so relieved she or he won't
even notice what you eat. (And if you're the one supposed to
be cooking, nobody will take offence anyway.)

You can go for a longer walk before you go to bed – or
walk part of the way home now, or both.

And tomorrow you can do your very best to eat as little
as possible until the evening so your body gets the benefit
of a partial "fast".

Or vow only to have 500 calories for the whole time
you're awake so it gets a full one.

In the meantime, you take some deep breaths and calm yourself. Probably by now your brain has registered all that sugar and has sent a "Yuck! Overload!" message to your stomach and if you just stop and listen to both of them you'll realise you don't want any more biscuits, in fact you're rather wishing you'd only had two.

So you get a grip. It's one bout of over-indulgence. Tomorrow is another day. Nobody has died. Etc.

And remember that you can eat a *lot* of food and get away with it if you only shift yourself too.

So let's have a little tiny square of chocolate, and get on to that –

20 WAYS TO FIGHT THE FLAB WITH EXERCISE

Yes, of course, the simple alternative to the whole of the above is to eat what you like, when you like, but exercise like a mad thing day and night.

Not many of us have time to do that but if you employ a combination of tactics – try some of the food-based strategies suggested and also shift yourself to the extent you can manage – you will really see a difference.

Exercise makes us feel good and builds muscle. Muscles, historically, burn more calories than fat (though some experts have begun disputing this and saying the difference is negligible. Let's not listen to them!) so there is an argument for not being restrictive as to what you take in so much as ensuring you burn it all off.

This is all very well if you have lots of hours available to go to the gym, run marathons, attend Bums & Tums classes (and can stomach the woman – there is always one – who has a perfect physique and just comes to preen on one leg and share with the lesser mortals the enviable sight of her admirably-sculptured, lycra-clad buttocks. Grr.) or swim sixty lengths of the local pool.

But if, actually, you have things like a life or a job or children and free minutes are at a premium, quick bursts of activity will work well too. These are things you can do that are cheap and easily fitted in.

1 Get a dog.

I have noticed that a lot of people who should, by rights, be fatter than they are, have a mutt that they walk through rain and shine. I am more of a cat person. I find dogs too time-consuming, too needy, and too fond of licking their testicles and then wanting to do the same to my face. I am also squeamish about picking up warm poo. But there is no doubt at all that talking regular brisk walks is an excellent way of keeping the weight under control and one's thighs and bum toned.

2 Borrow a dog.

This is a good compromise. I enjoy taking out Kenzo, a black Labrador belonging to my friend Lyn-Marie and Kenzo and I have an arrangement. He does a poo in the garden before we leave and I take him to all the muddy places he's not usually allowed. I also have an arrangement with Lyn-Marie. Should Kenzo ever let me down, I will phone her on her mobile and she will send one of the children to clear up.

My fondness for dog-walking (if not ownership) is probably what attracted me to the competition entry from Cathy Lennon, whose top flab-fighting tip made her another runner-up prize in the Fight the Flab competition:

Acquire a Labrador by Cathy Lennon.

"The canine equivalent of the fat bridesmaid in lemon taffeta on your wedding photos, a Labrador will do comparative wonders for your silhouette. But he's a practical help as well. You can get rid of those kitchen scales – when it comes to

portion control, what he can demolish in thirty seconds makes
the contents of your plate seem positively dainty. Even better,
your chances of finishing anything are slim. Without a lifebelt
and wellies, you'll have to hand over at least half of what
you're eating or risk drowning in a drool tsunami. Not only
can the Labrador deploy the Vulcan death stare to Oscar-
winning standard when you're trying to eat, he will offer you
the same 'aid to willpower' when it comes to exercise.
Labradors are creatures of habit. You thought death and taxes
were hard to avoid? Try missing his usual walk time ..."

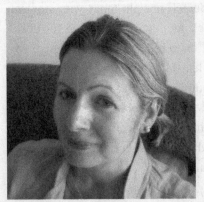

https://twitter.com/clenpen

3 Borrow a horse.

This could be more complicated to arrange but horse riding
will also give you muscles of iron. I have this problem
licked ever since begging for and receiving a hilarious
Christmas present which had my husband choking over his
credit card statement for the next six months. The ijoy ride
is an exercise machine that simulates the action of riding a
horse and as you jog up and down, tones your buttocks,

thighs and stomach. You can flap your arms at the same time, add weights, and do various exercises as outlined in the DVD of suitably bored-looking girls that comes with it. Visiting children will enjoy it too. Plonk the smallest and loudest on there and turn it up to full speed before they can trash the place.

4 Sit on a ball.

One of those exercise balls that you inflate. In a similar vein to the vibrating horse, the idea is that you wobble away and the effort of keeping yourself upright tones your stomach muscles, firms your backside, etc. I can vouch for this. I spent a week balanced on a big one while I typed. My stomach definitely felt less blobby by the end of it, but I found I was tending to support myself via my wrists on the desk after a while and gave myself sore shoulders. So perhaps watch TV on it instead – causing great hilarity throughout the family when you get carried away clapping along to *X Factor* and fall off.

5 Go for a run.

A good pair of trainers (and a sturdy bra for the girls) and you're off. Even if you just run up the road and back or once round the car park, you will boost your metabolism and burn calories. You will also tone up all over but particularly on your legs and bum. If you force yourself up hills, the effect on the latter can be remarkable. Some personal trainers believe that the best time to run – or do any exercise – is first thing in the morning before you've eaten. Particularly if the run or work-out will last less than thirty minutes.

Running on an empty stomach will maximise fat-burning and, unless you have an underlying health condition, you should be able to trot round the block without fainting. When I am in a running phase (this hasn't happened for a while) I also like to ring the changes and go at six o'clock. This has an unwinding effect after a hard day bashing away at the keyboard, the release of endorphins during physical activity leaving one clear-headed and relaxed for the evening ahead. It also means one can feel perfectly justified in having a gin and tonic and a bowl of peanuts.

6 Jump on a trampoline.

If the kids have got a big one in the garden so much the better but otherwise get yourself a trampette (also known as an aerobic bouncer or a rebounder) – one of those mini circular jobs – and leap up and down on that. You can jog, hop, or do star jumps – it will come with a leaflet with suggested exercises – and hold a small weight or a tin of baked beans in each hand to intensify the effect. It's quite good fun, kind on the joints, and a good way of burning calories and firming muscles. Just the two words of warning … both for the females. 1. Wear that sports bra and 2. If you've had children – they will laugh at you. If you've had lots of children, best have a wee before you start …

7 Do press-ups, squats and sit-ups.

You could try to get into the habit of doing a few press-ups and/or sit-ups in the mornings or before you go to bed, or in front of *EastEnders*. They are, without doubt, dull and boring and – until your stomach muscles shape up – hard

153

work to boot. But they do work eventually and you will feel a new definition to that soft bit round your middle. And then think how pleased you'll be when it's time to strip off for the beach.

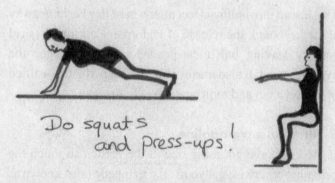

Do squats and press-ups!

When it comes to your rear end, there are a heap of different squat-type exercises you can find if you hit Google but here are a couple of basic ones. If you do just twenty of these each day (no, me neither, but get a grip and be a bit more disciplined), you will tone up your *derrière* in no time …

Method one: (avoid if you have dodgy knees) is to stand with your feet apart – beneath your hips – and then with your hands placed on your hips, slowly bend at the knees as if you were about to sit on a chair that's not there. Hold for a few seconds, rise and repeat. If you *have* got dodgy knees, they will probably drive you mad by clicking so best to do this one instead:

Method two: taught to me years ago by skiing friends who were going on the piste …

154

Stand against a wall with your feet apart, again to the width of your hips, and slowly slide your back down the wall until you are in a sitting position, with your feet about a foot away from the skirting board. Picture yourself on an imaginary chair and everything will be in the right place. Now hold that as long as you can. When you have recovered, do it again. It is much harder than it sounds, hurts quite a lot, quite soon, but will give you rock-hard thighs and a toned bottom.

What is more fun is to:

8 Go up and down stairs on your bottom.

Like a child might. I can offer no scientific evidence that this tones you up but it certainly feels as if it does. Try it and feel how many muscles are working! I have just practised it for you half a dozen times and I'm exhausted. If you can do it without using your arms, it's even more strenuous. (Please, however, be careful and do not fall down the stairs and then attempt to sue me.) If you cannot imagine what I'm talking about there are instructional videos on YouTube. (Of course.)

9 Use the stairs whenever you can.

If you can swap the lift or escalator for a few flights of the real thing, do so.

If you work from home, work upstairs.

Running downstairs every time you want to raid the fridge will burn fat and using stairs generally is great for legs and bottoms. So run up and down them anyway. The winter our heating was on a go-slow and I huddled in the kitchen all day as my office was arctic, I soon saw the difference. Not in a good way.

10 Use a pedometer.

A few years ago there was an NHS campaign to encourage us all to walk 10,000 steps a day and pedometers were being given away on the back of cornflakes packets. Interested to see how many steps I actually did clock up in a day, I bought one around that time and added counting my steps to my collection of small obsessions. I still walk round with what is now about my fifteenth pedometer (they get dropped, lost, broken, or trodden on at an alarming rate) clipped to my waistband and attempt to do 70,000 steps a week (my average is 56,000). It serves as a good indicator of whether one is moving enough (I have been sitting at this computer for hours) and helps with target-setting. If I've had a particularly sedentary day I can resolve to do better tomorrow or do that trot round the block.

If I'm feeling especially OCD and it's raining outside, I can pace the bedroom till the magic number is met, or run up and down the stairs. I think it keeps me fit. My son thinks I am being "sad".

11 Use your local shops.

Walking there will burn calories. Carrying the shopping home will tone arms some more. And if you are lucky enough to live near a proper High Street with small independent shops, you'll be helping the local economy and socking one in the eye to the supermarkets too. Multi-tasking for the Green and Ethical.

12 Walk on squishy soles.

I've long been a fan of Masai Barefoot Trainers. They cost a fortune but are supposed to mimic the action of walking on soft sand or similar, thus burning up three times the calories expended in ordinary footwear and getting rid of cellulite to boot. If ever there was a divide between the sexes, nothing highlights it like these shoes. When I first got them, men invariably guffawed condescendingly while women all but mugged me. I'm probably fortunate in my genes because I have never suffered from the orange peel stuff, but within weeks of first wearing MBTs I could see my legs were definitely more toned and my husband even told me my bottom looked smaller. (He is not a man to whom you ask "Does my bum look big in this?" unless you really want to know). The trainers (or sandals for summer) come with a DVD showing you how to walk in them. (Basically you keep your shoulders over your hips, roll the foot, and don't thrust your pelvis out until you can move without weaving about.) Might feel like hard work at first but worth it.

13 Drink, don't drive.

Don't ever take your car out with you in the evenings. Or quite enough cash for a cab. That way you will be forced to walk home (or at least back from the bus stop) and will expend lots of energy before you get to bed. NB I know I am banging on about walking A LOT but doing lots of it really does make a difference. My new friend, the ultra-charming[7] Zacchary Falconer-Barfield, lost 5kg in three months by simply adding walking to his routine. He now walks 4–8 miles a day. "Walking is just as good for you as pretty much any other cardio," he says, "but not so harmful on the knees." Zach tries

Footnote 7 Check him out on www.theperfectgentleman.tv

to do two sessions a day – "a long one first thing in the morning and a short one at night" (that's my boy!), and says: "the benefits are tremendous but on top of that you get to see where you live in a different light. If you live in a city like I do, you might find a secret alleyway or a new restaurant!"

Zacchary is therefore a role-model for us all. Brisk-walking his way to a flab-free world, while keeping an eye out for fab places to eat!

Rock on.

14 Tone your arms.

Even thin people with flabby arms don't look as good as bigger people with biceps of steel. Toned arms look fantastic, and distract from a multitude of other sins. If your upper arms are firm and you've successfully dealt with that floppy bit under the armpit you are going to look great in anything – and the world is your oyster when it comes to sleeves and off-the-shoulder. If you're a young thing in your twenties and thirties there'll be admiring glances galore. If you are over forty, nobody will even notice the size of your backside, they'll be too busy crowding round to ask how you did it. If you're over fifty – you'll be a legend!

Some toning methods that work:

Put all the nice food in very high cupboards. The constant stretching up will work wonders.

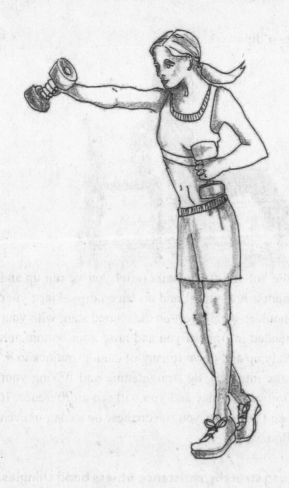

Punch with weights. I've got some of those weights with handles. They aren't particularly heavy – 3kg each – but if you shadow box with them for a few minutes a day, it really does help to tone up your upper arms. It can also help, on occasion, to calm one down. Simply imagine that instead of punching thin air, you are giving all who've done you wrong a damn good pasting …

Do tricep dips

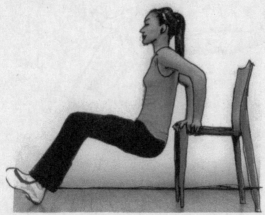

Sit on the bottom of the stairs (after you've run up and down them a few times) and do tricep dips. Place your hands shoulder-width apart on the second stair, with your legs extended in front of you and raise your bottom and upper body up and down (plenty of demonstrations to be had on the internet), by straightening and flexing your arms. Do twenty a day and you will see a difference. If you haven't got stairs, you can do these on a chair or even on the floor.

Buy those stretchy, resistance fitness band thingies.
Or whatever they're called. Get a couple and keep one in your pocket or handbag and one where you can see it while you work. Whenever you have a spare moment – waiting for the train, in the post office queue, while the potatoes are boiling or emails downloading, you can whip it out and do a few exercises. Just wrapping the band round a knee or foot and pulling it back and forth will give your bingo wings

something to think about but there are lots of exercises on the internet – with demonstrations on YouTube to help you focus specifically on triceps and wobbly bits.

Buy cheap cooking utensils.
The sort of scrubbing a bargain baking tray will need after a single roast will give arms a work-out.

Swim keeping your legs still.
If you do have time to visit the local pool, try a few lengths of breast stroke using only your arms with your legs held straight out behind you. Not difficult but intensifies the workout. You can alternate this with lengths using only using your legs – arms held straight in front of you, hands clasped. A little trickier but you won't drown. (NB as long as you can swim in the first place.)

Be arm aware.
Think arms whatever you do. Tense them and put extra effort into anything that involves your biceps and triceps. Can you feel the muscles tightening as you wield that corkscrew?

Arm wrestle.
After all that, you'll probably win.

15 Try the power plate.
If you belong to a gym, they'll have one there. I have found doing press-ups on this vibrating wonder machine quite dramatic in the firming up department and there are easy-to-

follow exercises for all parts of the body. (I will be very grown-up and won't make the joke obvious about sitting on it.) If you are rich, you could get one for home use. If you aren't, you could go to a sports equipment store and pretend you are. Ask for a full demonstration of their most expensive model and to try it yourself for half an hour while you think about it. Go back the next day in a different wig and do it again.

Since discovering the power of the power plate I have actually given up my gym membership and bought a vibrating plate thing, vastly reduced on the internet, with the money I am going to save over six months. It took all afternoon, much swearing, and copious alcohol to put it together, but it is a lot easier to exercise now I've got one downstairs rather than a drive away.

16 Keep your favourite foods in the loft.
Climbing up and down the ladder every time you fancy some cheese & onion crisps will tone your thighs in no time.

17 Tie a string round your waist.
Or a nice classy piece of ribbon. It acts as an aide-memoire to remind you to hold your stomach muscles in. There are a hundred exercises you can do to tighten your abs – sit-ups and press-up for example as mentioned earlier – but simply holding your muscles in and keeping them there is the simplest and the one you can do anywhere (a bit like pelvic floor squeezes but these make me squeamish). Stand up and draw your stomach muscles in so your waist circumference visibly shrinks. Then tie your string around your newly-narrowed middle – not so tightly it cuts off your circulation

obviously, but so that you feel the pull of it when you forget and let it all hang out again. I am of course trialling this for you – all these tips are exhaustively tried and tested (with the possible exception of the great sex) – and have now been holding my stomach muscles in for half an hour. The idea is that eventually they will do it all on their own without me thinking about it. I don't think they are quite ready to yet.

18 Get on your bike.

If you've got a bike you don't use, dust off the cobwebs and get pedalling, or consider acquiring one. Cycling burns anything from 180 to 400 calories an hour, uses all the major muscles in the lower body, burns fat – especially if you apply the principles of interval training to it – cycle fast for a minute, slow down for two etc. – and is kind to joints. There are cycling fitness programmes you can look up on the internet (Matt Roberts is always a good name to look out for, for any kind of get-fit or personal training advice) and older people can enjoy riding a bike as much as the kids. It gets you out in the fresh air, if you get a rack or a pannier you can pick up a bit of shopping at the same time, and it's a chance to look nosily into other people's gardens in a manner that's just not possible when driving a car.

19 Dance!

Dancing is great. It's aerobic, feel-good, and uses around 300 calories an hour depending on how vigorously you throw yourself around. You can go to classes but if you don't mind the sniggers of any passing offspring, it's just as easy to do it at home with the music blasting through the house or your earphones in. It is also useful as a bargaining tool for recalcitrant teenagers. If they don't tidy their room/pick up the towels/remove that festering plate from beneath the sofa, you will be shaking your body to the strains of Madonna's "Like a Virgin" when their friends come round.

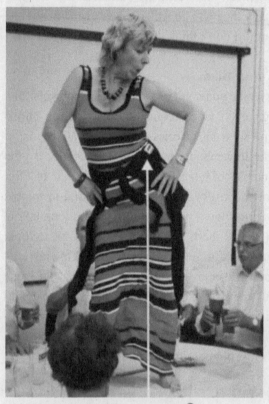

Note small obsession with pedometer;
see Excercise Tip no.10

Dance! But not necessarily on the table …
Photo by Bill Harris

20 Do something each day.

Your lifestyle and personal circumstances will not necessarily lend themselves to doing any of the above regularly, or indeed at all. But the important thing is to do *something*. Because you can eat a lot more if you do. And you are more likely to keep an activity up if you enjoy it, so try a few things out. Some people adore Zumba, others find their niche in a pilates class – you might be enthused by bowls or badminton.

I came to badminton and tennis quite late but I love them both so much (I make up with enthusiasm what I lack in ability) that it is never a chore to go and play and I would do it every day if time and available partners permitted. My policy is to make sure I do some sort of calorie-burning activity every day, even if I've got deadlines coming out of my ears and can only manage a power walk to the post box. Or if it's blowing a gale and pouring with rain and I'm feeling a wimp, then I'll at least do some exercises on the floor or have a jump on my mini trampoline.

If you want to keep on top of the flab, promise yourself you'll try to do some sort of exercise every single day, too. You'll be boosting your metabolism, toning your muscles, doing your heart good, and lowering your stress levels. And giving yourself a hell of a lot more scope to eat cake.

NB And the good news from the experts is that these days, exercise has got quicker! The latest thinking is that you can make quite a significant difference to your fitness in quite a short time per day – so even ten minutes devoted to a few exercises will pay dividends.

What works best is interval training – bursts of intense

activity followed by a short period of rest, then more intense activity. You may like to check out *Fast Exercise* a book by Michael Moseley (of the fasting fame) and the health and fitness journalist, Peta Bee, which looks at getting and keeping fit in only a few minutes of workout each day.

And if it's only a few minutes you've got: our third runner-up in the Fight the Flab competition – Tony Tibbenham – has provided this top exercise tip.

Roll 6 for chocolate.

"If you really want that chocolate, roll a dice and if you get a 6, you are allowed the treat. Variations include rolling two dice and only granting yourself the treat if they both land on 6 and you get the double. But for maximum benefit, roll really vigorously, so you are forced to scramble all over the room, over chair and beneath sofa, to retrieve the dice. That way you get exercise too."

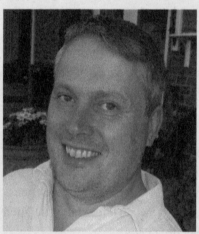

photo by Jane Wenham-Jones

DRESSING UP, SIZING DOWN

25 ways to *look* thinner, even if you're not ...

1 Posture is everything.

However much you weigh, you'll look a whole lot leaner
with a straight back. If you have a tendency to shuffle along
staring at your feet or standing in a slump with your
stomach hanging out, stop now. Place yourself in front of a
mirror and stand tall. Relax your shoulders, hold your head
erect and look where the horizon would be. See the
difference? Now stay like that. And walk like it too.

2 Wear the right clothes.

If you are built like a manikin, anything you wear, from
three knotted hankies to a Tesco carrier bag, will look good.

This is why the manikins in shop windows have waists the
circumference of the average woman's thigh. And why the
whole look of a garment can alter drastically if we put on, or
lose, weight. Having said that, it is also perfectly possible to
look seven pounds heavier or lighter just by thinking carefully
about the way you dress. Compare and contrast, for example,
your appearance when slobbing out at home in a pair of
shapeless tracksuit bottoms and a washed-out T-shirt – tucked
in – with how you look in your most punishing hold-it-all-

back underwear, fitted dress and perilous heels (or for you more conservative chaps, a well-cut suit!).

A lot of it is down to choosing attire in an enhancing shape and cut, in the right fabric, flattering colour and to a good fit. That's the aesthetics but there's more. The thing about wearing the right clothes is that if they *are* right, they will make you feel good. And once you look in the mirror and you like what you see, you will have confidence. If you have confidence, you'll relax and feel happy. And if you feel happy you'll look terrific. Simple. Never mind how much extra flesh you've got.

If you are like me, this magic combination can be a bit of a moveable feast. I am incapable of travelling light because I can never be sure which clothes are going to make me feel good on any particular day so I always have to carry a choice. But if you know the sort of thing that works for you and can follow a few general rules, then you have a better chance of cutting to the chase.

My friend Janice, who knows a bit about fashion and used to style brides, actually has a bigger waist than I do but looks much tinier. She puts this down to clever upholstery. She pays as much attention to what goes on underneath as what you see on top and it works like a charm. Janice believes in petticoats (for a smooth finish and no unsightly lines), good cuts, and what she calls "Harvest Festival Knickers" – where all has been safely gathered in.

3 Wear big knickers.

Or whatever underwear it takes! You can buy brilliant undergarments these days that can totally revolutionise your shape. Why not let them? Look around the room at the next party. Half the people you see who look good are probably holding themselves together by this means.

I remember the night I met up with a good friend. She was wearing a skin-tight red, glittery number and not only looked fantastic but about three stone lighter than she had at lunchtime. "Where's your stomach gone?" I shrieked diplomatically, having seen her at large only hours before. She gave a secretive smile.

"I'm wearing one of those squash-it-all-in things," she confided. "If the poppers give way, it's every man for himself …"

I went straight out and bought one myself but I can advise that, like most things, some are better than others. You need it to be tight but also well cut. Some of the lesser examples of the all-in-one "body-shaper" send all the spare blubber into a nasty bulge that pops out under your arms or half way down your thighs. Make sure you are being flattened out evenly.

(To any chaps reading – this is not as irrelevant as you think – you can get male girdles too!)

A good rule of thumb is that if you can't breathe or sit down and going to the loo is out of the question, then it's probably working. NB If you are in the early stages of a relationship or hoping to land a new conquest, this is not the time to rush into things or let him undress you. If he does manage to wrest you from the garment in question, you'll probably knock him out.

4 Wear bigger knickers.

I once worked with a very thin and irritating girl who, if she spotted anyone daring to eat between meals, particularly anything more calorific than an alfalfa sprout, would wag a reproving finger and chant "Pickers wear bigger knickers …"

I would say sensible females wear them too. If I can give you one decent tip on looking good in your clothes it is to always buy your pants one size larger than your dress size. Nothing looks worse than VPL (visible panty line for the uninitiated) and it causes even really slim women to instantly appear podgier. If your knickers are roomy they will lie comfortably flat against your skin and not create any unsightly bulges. Perhaps this is just my little foible but if it goes viral remember you heard it here first.

5 Look to the stars.

This is another Janice tip. Search for the celebrity who most matches your body shape and size and who you think looks particularly good. Then Google image them and copy their style. (Be sensible, says Janice. Don't aim to look like Uma Thurman when you naturally look more like Dawn French.) As Janice points out, stars often use style consultants, so you may as well benefit vicariously from their professional advice.

6 Don't look to size zero.

Remember when Kylie went on tour in a corset that reduced her waist to sixteen inches? It brought forth a rash of "hourglass" diets. Go fetch a tape measure, bend it into a circle and see what a waist of sixteen inches looks like. Inhuman! There is no point aspiring to that. Go look at the dimensions of Victoria Beckham in Madame Tussards. There is no point in aspiring to that either. Unless you look like that naturally which you probably don't. (Or why would you be reading this?)

Stay real.

7 Find your USP (unique selling point).

What's your best feature? Accentuate it! If it's your eyes, wear a colour that brings them out. If it's your cleavage, flaunt it, if you've got long legs, wear clothes that show them off. Who'll have time to think about your stomach and backside?

8 If you know you're going to eat, dress accordingly.

If you are going somewhere where you know there'll be copious food and drink – a wedding, say, or dinner at the friends who always serve five courses, then you will not want to be wearing the equivalent of a corset. Instead wear clothes that are roomy around the middle but still disguise the worst of the bulge. A-line dresses that are fitted around the bust can work well and look sexy. Or if you're really going to pork out – a flowing top over elasticated trousers.

9 Employ cardigans and light jackets.

To disguise lumps and bumps from the sides but still show off a curvy shape from the front. If the front is a problem too, try a dangling scarf. Or a poncho.

10 Never tuck anything in.

Not unless you're wearing that jacket.

11 Ignore labels.

When buying clothes, never be swayed by anything it says on the label (unless it's "dry-clean only"). Only focus on what it looks like. Clothes on the large side look infinitely better than anything too tight and it is madness to squeeze yourself into an unflattering 14 because you refuse to acknowledge the 16 fits. You can lose the tag later.

Even if something appears to fit, it is worth trying on the size below and size above. An over-sized jumper can look great over tight jeans and sometimes, despite one's fears, a closer-fitting dress can be more flattering.

If it's an important occasion you're shopping for, take a friend who can be relied on to be brutal. Take the shoes you'll wear with you – and possibly the big knickers ensemble too. I am a size 10-12. The clothes in my wardrobe range from size 8-16 and I wear them all. If the label upsets me, I cut it out.

And then lie about it.

12 Ditch the fat clothes.

By this, I don't mean the clothes you wear on a fat day – we all need to keep a few billowing things for then – but the clothes that make you look fatter than you need to. I have a bright green dress in a great design that looks fabulous on the hanger. It might look good on you too. On me it adds ten pounds. (There is a photo of me in it floating about the internet which pops up from time to time – ugh. But at least it's a good incentive.)

I keep the dress out of interest to see what it will look like when, one day, I go on the weight-loss plan of my life and end up weighing seven and a half stone (that is 105 pounds to my American cousins – no, not very likely is it?), but I should just give it away now. Life is too short to wear clothes that do not make you look the best you can. Go through your wardrobe with a weather eye or a good friend and fill that charity sack.

If you do get thin, you'll want new clothes anyway.

13 Learn from the slimming clothes.

Look at the clothes that do make you look good and analyse them. Make a note of the shape and length and cut of your favourite, most flattering garments and go shopping with that in mind. If something has immediately sprung to mind, write it down in the box below, before you forget again. At the same time, don't forget what doesn't work. I've learned I cannot wear three-quarter length sleeves, and bought at least three little denim jackets to wear over summer dresses before it finally sunk in that I can't wear them without looking ghastly. Now I wear a certain shape of cardigan instead. If you've got things in your wardrobe which were a big mistake, write notes on those down too, to save you buying something similar.

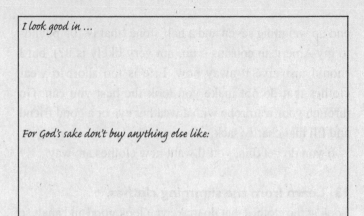

I look good in …

For God's sake don't buy anything else like:

14 And wear them even at home.

We've all got stuff we slob about in at home that is not for public consumption but it helps if even these garments are ones you feel good about yourself in.

If you live in T-shirts and tracksuit bottoms choose ones that flatter your shape – I've got two lots of jogging bottoms that look identical on the face of it, except one pair gives me a flattish stomach and the other is downright depressing.

If you're wandering around in a floppy sundress make it the sort that covers a multitude of sins. If you have any sort of at-home ensemble that makes you look like a swollen bag person, for goodness' sake, go bin it now. Because if you catch sight of yourself in the mirror looking shapeless and lardy you will feel demoralised and more likely to overeat. If you look slim, you'll act slim – and that's half the battle. (Remember we are still Thinking Thin!)

But that's only *my* theory. Karen Booth, our next runner-up in the Flab-fighters' competition takes a different approach:

The Regulating Waistband Plan.

"Sort the contents of your wardrobe into two piles – one a size or two smaller than your real size, the other one or two sizes bigger than you really need (this shouldn't be a problem for anyone who can relate to yo-yo dieting who's likely to have a range of sizes in their wardrobe for fat and thin stages). The idea is to wear the smaller sizes whenever you're at home or working alone – anytime you're not going to come across many people. You'll find it difficult stuffing yourself when your waistband's cutting you in two, you're likely to feel full quicker and the rolls and muffin tops you see every time you pass a mirror will be a candid reminder of the need to watch what you eat! When it comes to socialising and being in company, it's time to choose from the 'two sizes bigger' outfits and revel in the compliments when your friends ask if you've lost weight – well surely you must have done, your clothes are hanging off you! This method also works well with the 'fast and feed' plan, wearing your tight clothes on fast days will leave you feeling like you've troughed your way through a five-course meal, whereas your bigger outfits on a feed day will allow you to feel comfortable eating what you like – just don't overdo it and end up filling your 'big' pants!"

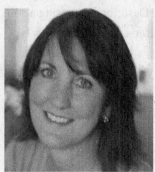

Karen Booth
http://thewritingbooth.blogspot.co.uk/

15 Put on white leggings.

Or some equally unflattering attire, with a T-shirt tucked in and stomach thrust out. That's how gross you could look. But you won't, will you, 'cos you're going to eat a chilli every day and go up and downstairs on your bottom. See what I can do for you? Now bin this stuff and follow point 14 on previous page.

16 Buy a Doreen.

I had never heard of one of these until Janice slipped me the word, but it is allegedly the UK's, if not the world's, best-selling bra! I got mine when I was in a play. It was Terrence Rattigan's *Separate Tables* and I was playing the forty-year-old ex-model Anne Shankland. Needless to say I went on an immediate diet – the last thing I wanted during my big moment was to hear someone muttering from the audience: *she looks a bit old and fat to be a model* ... and I consulted Janice re my costume. She packed me off to Debenhams post-haste and I have been a Doreen convert ever since. This bra, from Triumph, is one of those old-fashioned-looking garments of the sort your mum or granny used to wear – a sheepdog bra, as Janice puts it – that rounds them up and points them in the right direction. Described as having a soft cup, firm underband, and wide straps, it gives a fifties type silhouette and because your bust is hoiked up, it elongates your middle section between your ribs, which is very slimming. Whenever I wear my Doreen under a close-fitting top or dress, I am asked if I've lost weight. I like that.

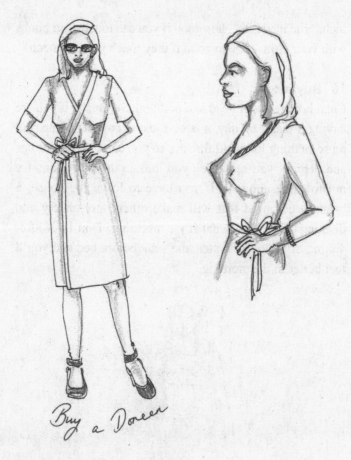

Buy a Doreen

17 Make sure your bra fits.

Janice is evangelical on the subject of brassieres and it is
true that a good bra makes all the difference to your overall
look – there is nothing worse than overspill or under-hang
or bulges beneath the arms. It is really worth getting a
proper fitting and spending time making sure you've got the
right bra for the right outfit (sports bras are for sport, sniffs
Janice). "For special occasions shorten bra straps inch by

inch," she instructs. "It is good if you can touch your boobs with your chin – not so good if they touch your stomach!"

18 Buy a tent.

Cut a hole for your head and put it on. Seriously, if you are having a really fat day, it is best just to cover it all up. Put on something long and flowing so you can't see the lumps and depress yourself when you look in the mirror and try not to think about it. If you have to leave the house, a brightly coloured tent will make others feel cheery and distract them from what it's concealing. Don't eat after 4 p.m., drink lots of water, and walk before bed and you'll feel better in the morning.

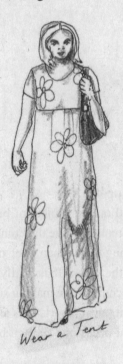

Wear a Tent

19 Wear heels.

Not all the time obviously – but whenever you want to create an extra illusion of slimness and elegance. "Court shoes elongate the leg," says Janice. "Ankle straps are sexy but tend to shorten it." (I don't know as I rarely wear shoes, preferring boots.) Can I also suggest that you either wear a short skirt or a long skirt. Unless you have very thin legs, mid-calf promotes the tree-trunk look. This applies to both sexes.

20 With support tights.

No wonder Spanx as a company is now worth over a billion dollars. Support tights – particularly Spanx – work nothing short of a miracle on stomachs and waists and bottoms. Even if you have to allow an extra twenty minutes to get them on. They do not come cheap but what price a nipped-in middle when you need one. Other companies (including M&S) do their own reasonably-priced versions. For best effect combine with a Doreen (see earlier). And cut your nails first – nothing worth than finally getting them on, putting yourself in the recovery position and then spotting the ladder from knee to ankle …

21 Choose great swimwear.

If you're going to reveal your bikini body, invest in good gear. Firm cups give shape, Ruching can be good – no one knows what's fabric and what's you – and psychedelic colours can blind the onlooker to what's beneath. Chaps – be sensible. Tiny teeny swimming trunks? Not unless you are seven years old. And quite frankly, even then …

22 Wear statement jewellery.

Massive earrings, huge nose studs, or something quirkily-shaped round your neck will, I am quite sure, distract the eye from your stomach …

23 Watch the camera.

The proliferation of camera phones is a scourge of our times and I am fed up with lardy photos of me popping up on Facebook. Not much you can do about that but un-tag them pronto and give the "photographer" a roasting when you next see him/her. But when you are aware of what is going on, there are a few simple precautions you can take. When photographed in a group, don't stand on the end. Bulldoze your way into the middle, put your arm around the shoulders of the person either side of you and hide your fat bits behind them. When pictured on your own, hold your arms away from your body, suck in your stomach – see above – and then find someone good with PhotoShop.

24 Buy tummy tuck jeans.

These clever trousers, also known as Not Your Daughter's Jeans are not your regular legwear – the range has been specially designed to flatten your tummy and lift your bottom.

You buy these unlikely garments several sizes smaller than you would usually contemplate (I squeezed myself into a UK size four!) and prepare to be amazed. One looks at a size smaller at least – and somehow taller – yet once you've had them on for half an hour, the stretchiness makes them as comfortable as leggings. The price might take your breath away but boy, are they worth it. Mine are black with sparkly bits but they come in different colours. If you saw them on the hanger and then looked me up and down you'd never believe I could get them on. (After sitting for a week at this computer, I'm not sure I do either.)

25 Pretend you weigh much more than you do.

Most of us shave a bit off our weight when we're talking to others, but the reverse works much better. Announce gaily that you weigh fourteen stone, when you really weigh nine and you will be met with gasps of disbelief and admiration.

"Gosh you don't look it," they will cry. "You must have lead toes," they may shriek. You will be instantly admired for your ingenious way with clothes and the clear evidence that you must be "big-boned" or "all muscle". If you do things the other way round, there will a shaking of heads and some pointed staring at your spare tyre. The same principle applies to lying about your age and wrinkles.

IF YOU NEED TO
SHIFT IT FAST

Losing masses of weight in a very short space of time is not generally to be recommended. I confess I have never truly understood why and experts don't necessarily agree on the pros and cons either.

But theories put forward includes the notion that any rapid loss will be mostly water and could even be lean tissue to boot; that fat cells are used by the body to store toxins – such as those from pesticides and pollutants – and if we lose weight quickly they get flooded back into our blood streams; that on a very low-calorie regime we may not be getting all the essential nutrients we need (a low intake of iron and calcium can be a particular problem); and most of all, because if we lose weight very fast, it is apparently much more likely to go back on quickly as well.

All I can contribute on a personal level is some anecdotal evidence that you can sweat for a fortnight to lose three pounds only to put it back on overnight after a few sandwiches and one good curry.

Having said all that, there are times when we want to lose weight quickly – usually before some big event for which we'd rather not be flashing too many spare tyres.

Can I first offer the obvious advice, which is to try not to *need* to shift it fast, but to start early? If there's one truism

I have finally grasped as I've got older it's that time whizzes past at an alarming rate and anything you undertake is always going to take longer to do than you think it will.

So while it is very easy to think that since the holiday isn't till August, there's no need to start worrying about your diet till June – after all if you lose weight too soon, you'll only put it back on etc. – there is actually every reason to start as soon as you can.

Because the fat might not start shifting as quickly as you hoped, events will conspire against you, you'll put your head in the sand, there will be parties and cake and offers on from the local take-away and you'll put it all off telling yourself there is plenty of time until you realise that to meet your target you have to lose ten pounds by next Wednesday.

I can't tell you how many times I have had big nights on the calendar for six months, made a mental note to lose just a couple of pounds a month till then (and how hard can that be? I have asked myself) and still waddled along on the night the exact same weight I was when I got the invitation …

Which is why this section exists: If you do need to look thinner in perilously few days' time you have to go at the challenge with gusto. I'm not usually a proponent of the somewhat blithe "eat less, move more" school of weight loss because I think it ignores the basic problems of feeling hungry and one's sense of deprivation that I held forth on at the very start, but in this instance, in the short term, you need to do just that.

If I'm trying to shed pounds in a hurry, I survive on spiced-up soup (my chillies again!) and tins of tuna served with a load of salad and a blob of mayonnaise. I favour a high protein approach because that staves off the worst of the hunger, but if I am hungry I tell myself that means the diet is working.

If you do this you will definitely lose weight:
- Eat a small protein breakfast – like my quick egg dish with some chilli in it – to get the metabolism going early.
- For the other meals, eat lean protein with salad and vegetables.
- Don't drink alcohol – or if that's a step too far, have a shot of gin or vodka with lots of slimline tonic and lemon and make it last.
- Drink lots of water.
- Do as much exercise as you can cram in. Walk and move as rapidly as possible in between.
- If you need a snack, have a small piece of cheese, a few nuts, or a square or two of very dark chocolate. Otherwise stave off hunger with hot drinks like herbal or green teas, the odd black coffee, and lots of positive thinking …
- The night before your big day if you can go to bed hungry you will wake up with a much flatter stomach.

Good things to tell yourself when ready to gnaw the bedpost:
- *I am feeling ravenous because my body is burning up fat.*
- *It is not a feeling I am going to die of.*
- *I will soon have forgotten this feeling I have now, but*

184

the photos of me tomorrow could be on Facebook for ever.

- *I will be hugely pleased with myself tomorrow when I am feeling slimmer and it will all have been worth it.*
- *I will not be a wuss.*

Then put a hot water bottle on your stomach, read a book, listen to the radio, and try to get to sleep early so you're oblivious to the pangs. You will be **so** glad you did …

PARTY WEEKS

Once you are actually at your party, feeling suitably small-stomached, taut-bottomed, and pleased with yourself, you want to have a good time.

And if you have any sort of life, there'll be other days and weeks when it is not convenient or pleasant to be stressing about your diet.

If you are travelling, going out a lot, staying with friends, or required to attend a big celebration, you don't want to be standing there clutching your plastic box full of carrot sticks, preparing to open your flask of low-cal celery gruel, when everybody else is necking back the champagne and cheese straws.

Or not without feeling deprived, stressed, and being a bloody nuisance, anyway.

For let us not forget that, unless you have an allergy that will render you dead on the floor if you accidentally eat a prawn or a peanut, then it is, anyway, rude to poke and pick.

The woman you've gone to dinner with may have been worrying about it for three days. For all you know, she's had a domestic, had to bribe the kids to sod off to bed without tantrums, and is only smiling because she hit the gin at 6 p.m.

The last thing she needs is you going into meltdown in

case there's hydrogenated fat in the cheesecake base. Smile, eat, be appreciative, and sort it out tomorrow.

And if you know you're headed for a few days of over-indulgence, you simply have to plan accordingly. If the food's going to be coming from all directions and you know the temptation will be all too much, then don't beat yourself up about that pudding but take steps (literally!) to minimise the damage.

I am writing this section on my return from the marvellous Chez-Castillon (check it out on www.chez-castillon.com) where the food is amazing, the wine flows (boy, does it flow) and I eat three meals a day plus crisps. (Betty Orme, another regular there I've mentioned earlier, shares my small salt weakness and Janie Millman, who, together with her husband Mike Wilson, runs the joint, indulges us with a bowl of nibbles of the deep-fried potato variety at regular intervals.)

I missed having breakfast proper a few mornings (because I was getting ready to teach) and only ate a tiny piece of a croissant or the small knob end of a French stick in haste on my way to the classroom, but apart from that I filled my boots.

There were no scales, but I can always tell from the mirror whether I'm putting it on – it goes straight to my stomach – and while there were a couple of mornings when I discerned a bit of a protuberance in my middle region (possibly after the day Katie Fforde and I flew back to England to attend über literary agent Carole Blake's Fifty Years in Publishing party, and we ate carbs *all* day – finishing off in the hotel bar with a grand dinner of a glass of Rioja each and a large of portion of chips!) I seemed to be doing OK. When I got home I confirmed that I had arrived back at exactly the same weight as I'd gone out there.

How?

Like this:

I walked. Author Catherine Jones (ex-army – favourite expression "Brace up") was training for a sponsored walk and she and I went on a brisk route march each afternoon for about an hour. We walked at a good rate and included a hill or two. (Sometimes she forced me up the same one twice).

I ran up and down the stairs. My room was two flights up – I went up and down with as much speed as I could muster unless I was carrying a cup of tea.

I took a turn round the block before bed most nights.

If I was going to go over the top on the scrumptious French bread I did it at lunchtime rather than the evening. At dinner I'd just have a little bit so I wouldn't feel I was missing out. And I have to say the cuisine is all good stuff. Janie creates brilliant salads (see recipe section), she uses fresh ingredients, and everything – even down to the delicious ice cream (I eat desserts here too!) – is homemade.

I sang (150 calories per hour), laughed (20% increase in calorie burning compared with sitting looking miserable) and danced (aerobic exercise that is fat-burning, and after all the alcohol I'd had, it needed to be).

And do you know what else I think helped? I was having a great time. I can't give you the science on this but remember what we said about the reason why people in love tend to lose weight? It's not just that they are concentrating on looking sexy and irresistible and don't want to ruin their sultry image by stuffing doughnuts, it's also because they are happy!

They skip about the place with a spring in their step rather than slumping on the sofa with a pork pie. Which uses up more energy and gives the metabolism a boost.

And thinking about it, you are more likely to be in that happy state if you determine that you won't be neurotic about your calorie intake but will enjoy yourself, have a damn good time, and mitigate the damage by doing some extra exercise. (Won't you?)

HOLIDAYS

Even if you are away for a fortnight, the same principles apply. Even when you are on an all-inclusive package and the buffet tables are groaning morning, noon, and night.

A few years ago I was a speaker on a cruise ship. I have never seen so much food in my life! It quickly became obvious that in the 12 days I was going to be aboard it would be perfectly possible to double one's girth. So after three days of feeling myself start to gently swell, I took decisive action.

I went brisk walking round the deck each morning (three circuits equalled a mile), I used the gym, I didn't use the lifts unless I was tottering in heels (cruises involve a lot of dressing up) and I had a small lunch if I knew I was going for the full six courses at dinner or a salad in the evening if I'd gone for afternoon tea.

By juggling it all around I had a really lovely time, ate and drank loads, and came back much the same on the weight front.

This is easier still, if you are staying somewhere where you can walk along the beach, swim, or play some sort of sport. Even if you prefer the sort of holiday where you remain horizontal, your only exercise the turning of the pages of your book or the lifting of cocktail glass to your lips, you may as well enjoy every minute of it. You can redress the balance when you get home and in the meantime, limit the worst of the podge-effect by possibly skipping the odd lunch or breakfast. You won't miss it in the whole scheme of things.

How to take off, without putting on ...

- Use the stairs where possible – if you are staying on floor ten of a hotel, you may not want or have time to walk all the way up, but you can do a couple of flights up and run some or all of the way down.
- Take the spicy option if you can. If necessary, carry your own little bag of dried chilli flakes and scatter them over whatever you're eating. (NB I am not talking desserts.)
- Drink lots of water
- Have a brisk walk before bed – even if it's only up and down those hotel stairs.
- If there's a chance for other exercise, take it.
- Then try to get enough sleep. As mentioned earlier, too few hours under the duvet can upset the hormones that govern hunger and lead those who are consistently sleep-deprived to gain weight. Make the most of the chance for a lie-in.

Have fun!

191

TONING AND TANNING

However much flesh you've got, there is no doubt it looks better brown. (NB this is not the same as orange). Even if you're going to be eating your body weight in cocktail snacks, a tan will still make you feel and look slimmer. And it's never been easier to get a fake one.

Though judging from some of the examples seen on parade, it is best to proceed with caution.

I have not tried an automatic tanning booth yet although friends seem pleased, but there are plenty of them about. I like having a tan done at home so I can wander around with almost no clothes on (you must wear loose garments afterwards). And I think the very best tans are achieved when the lotion is put on by hand and rubbed in to pre-scrubbed skin. But when the operator knows what she's doing, a spray is good too.

My lovely friend, Michaella Bolder, who is a tanner to the stars, has done both sorts for me and has set up a tanning booth in my kitchen – hilarious.

Even the do-it-yourself products are a lot more natural-looking and smell a lot less foul than they once did. Fake tanning yourself is OK to fill in strap marks or give your legs a quick boost – I like the St Tropez mousse you put on with a mitt – but I would never attempt any greater surface area without help – it's a bit difficult to do your own back! You may be braver.

But whether you do it yourself, with a friend or go to a salon, here are Michaella's hot top tanning tips just for you.

- Preparation is key for the perfect tan. Start by exfoliating and shaving/waxing 24 hours prior to tanning.
- Do not use perfume on the day of your tan and remove any deodorant from under your arms using an oil-free wet wipe. Moisturise dry areas – i.e. elbows, knees, hands and feet – using a body moisturiser
- If you are doing it yourself, use a mitt to apply the mousse or lotion. Apply the tan all over the body, making sure you bend the fingers and blend onto the hands and feet carefully, using what's on the mitt rather than adding product directly onto the skin.
- More is less. Don't be afraid to use a generous amount of product on the skin to ensure you cover all areas and no streaks are formed.
- Buff over the body once finished, with the last remains of product already on the mitt to even out the colour.
- Use a wet wipe to clean palms of hands and nails.
- Your tan must be left on the skin for at least 6-8 hours before getting the skin wet or showering.

I would like to add a piece of hard-won wisdom to the above: If you have a tan done just before you go on holiday – do not spend the first morning sitting on the edge of the pool with your legs immersed to mid calf while you read your book. By evening you will look as if you have been wearing socks. It is not a good look.

Tan and Tone

I have recently discovered a product called "Skinny Tan" which is supposed to do just that – the product combines fake tan and a cream designed to reduce the appearance of cellulite, thus making one appear skinnier, an innovation that had all the "dragons" scrabbling over it when it appeared on *Dragons' Den*. I wanted to try it out for you but Michaella and I were laughing so hysterically during her efforts to take before and after photos of my bottom that plans for an entire body treatment had to be abandoned. However the skin on the test area did feel quite soft and smooth and I thought maybe I detected that my bum was a tad more peachy. Michaella, down on her hands and knees inspecting it – the test of a true pal if ever there was one – said loyally that I didn't have any cellulite to start with (must be all that sisal sponging, MBT wearing, and running up and down the stairs). I would share the photos[8] so you could judge for yourselves, but they suffer from serious camera shake.

Footnote 8: I would also refer you to tip no 90.

FLAB-FIGHTING AT WORK

This flab-fighting business is all about being realistic and working round your lifestyle so if you have a long commute, have to get up early, go to bed late, work shifts, or have any number of reasons for being short on time to knock up perfectly balanced, calorie-controlled, nutrient-packed meals, and quite frankly are so knackered most evenings it's as much as you can do to wield the corkscrew and open a bag of peanuts — then some of the strategies suggested in this book may be beyond your energy levels or inclination.

And may I suggest that anyway, on weeks when you are *really* up against it, and already stressed to the eyeballs or under a lot of time pressure, that you don't worry too much about flab-fighting – except to make sure you are getting enough good food to give you the oomph and brain power to keep going. (B vitamins are good, as are omega 3-6-9 oils, so try to eat foods with these in or at least take them as supplements.)

Because the problem with cutting your calories simultaneously with chasing a deadline is that instead of focussing on your project, you are likely find yourself dreaming about cheese on toast or a bacon sandwich.

So you just have to do your best. And know that you can have a blitz on yourself next week, when you, say, eat lots of raw vegetables, cut down on your sugar, and get back into an exercise routine.

(NB unless, fellow writers – you are working on a book! In which case you daren't throw all caution to the winds for six months. Not unless you want a back end the size of Wiltshire – which is sort of where this all started.)

But I'm always busy, I hear you cry. "I'm always chasing deadlines." (*I AM writing a book*, comes the chorus from the already-expanding Writer's-Bottom brigade.) In that case you have to do what you can.

How to flab-fight when you're up against it.

Be really organised at the weekends. Plan menus or at least decide roughly the sort of things you're going to eat and fill the fridge and cupboards with foods that makes you happy and won't render you too gross. NB ready meals can be pretty good these days and most of the supermarkets do a totally-ready or easy-cook range made with decent ingredients that you can just stick in the oven the moment you walk in the door. Even if they are not officially "low calorie" or low fat, they will have all the nutritional information on the labelling so you can keep a weather eye on how much you're consuming in the evenings – if it's a lot, add a chopped chilli and get that brisk walk in. (If you've got a desk job, you need to be religious about finding time for some sort of physical activity.)

Make your own salad bar (or buy it in).

Make a big soup.

Prepare meals for the freezer.

Basically, do whatever it takes to ensure that there are good things to eat at home, so you are not tempted to have endless take-aways or bring back all the gooey, snacky stuff you can find that's on sale on the station.

Sometimes, if you get in late and you really feel very tired it's worth having a herbal tea – camomile is soothing and teapigs make the best – and just going to bed. You'll fall asleep before the hunger pangs become a problem and you'll feel lighter in the morning.

You'll also have the perfect excuse to indulge yourself at breakfast.

A WORD ABOUT
HOTEL BREAKFASTS

If you stay in hotels, for work or otherwise, you will know that being presented with a vast array of ready-prepared breakfast can be a challenge.

As a recent convert to the odd hearty start, I no longer worry about my self-restraint, but view the hot and cold buffet as a source of inspiration, not downfall.

As I see it, you are faced here with a very real chance of consuming 2000 calories before 10 a.m. and there are three ways in which you can approach this opportunity:

1) Eat everything in sight. Have strawberries and cereal, porridge and honey, the full cooked ensemble of eggs, bacon, sausage, black pudding, baked beans (if you can stomach the latter two – I'd prefer to munch my leg) and hash browns, toast, and croissants. Use the stairs not the lift and don't eat again till you have a tiny dinner. (You will get away with it.) And while you're enjoying every glorious morning mouthful, watch the thin girl – yes, that one with the sanctimonious expression who's clearly as miserable as sin and is spooning fat free yoghurt over her kiwi fruit. Do you want to be like that?

2) Sit piously sipping your green tea and nibbling on a blueberry (adopt a similar facial arrangement to the one you witnessed above) or your black coffee with a slice of cheese. Feel yourself bathed in self-righteous virtue and peruse the other guests.

See that fat family in the corner? The bloke with the stomach, who can barely move his plate, the annoying kids going back for more pastries? See how enormous his wife is?

Allow yourself a small sniff. That's why.

3) You remember that just because it's there you don't have to eat it. If you don't eat it, you'll have forgotten it by this evening.

If you do eat it, don't have lunch.

GIVE UP ON GUILT

Sometimes you'll overdo it, sometimes you won't. All I can say about anything I have suggested is: don't beat yourself up if it all goes wrong.

Because unless you are impossibly disciplined, annoyingly perfect and probably android, it will.

If to err is human then so is to eat too much.

By way of example, and solidarity, I will share with you the fact that at the time of writing this, I have just eaten three bags of crisps (yes – three!).

My family have gone away for a few days (hallelujah) and I have the house to myself in order to gain peace, quiet, and the chance to get this written.

When I got back from dropping them at the airport, I felt cross and uptight and anxious about the size of my to-do list and hungry and didn't fancy cooking or eating fruit (I do not find fruit mood-enhancing – you may do. If so, congratulate yourself, go eat some pomegranate and skip this bit where I admit to being a half-crazed carb-fuelled, out-of-control potential lard-arse. What am I doing writing a book like this anyway, you may well ask. Well quite. What are you doing, reading it?)

Anyway, there were grapes on the side but they weren't going to do it. Nor was a nice, well-chopped salad. I wanted fat and salt and possibly alcohol. So I'll tell you what I did.

I sat in my garden with a very large glass of pink fizz (probably one and a half "large" pub measures and enough to give whoever writes the government guidelines the vapours) and a bag of crisps tipped into a bowl (one does have standards). Then I replenished the crisps. Then I refilled my glass. Then I did the crisp thing again. How do I feel now? Very much better, thank you.

It would be easy to sink into a well of despair, fat-focussing and self-revulsion. But I am looking at it this way:

1) The bags were small. Each contained only 148 calories. Even taking into account that I ate three of them I have still only pigged out to the tune of 444 calories, plus the calories in the cava. I can have the salad for dinner and I can go for a brisk walk around the block before I go to bed. I am not going to put on even a pound – unless I now go into that aforementioned slough of despond and eat four doughnuts, some chips, and a lard sandwich. And as it happens, after the whole fat/salt/sugar combo of wine and crisps, I am quite fine having a jasmine tea and a small piece of chocolate. (As well as the salad, I can also have a vitamin pill.)

2) There was nothing terrible in there. The My-Body-Is-A-Temple brigade say "junk food' like they'd say 'heroin' but actually small slivers of potato cooked in sunflower oil is only that – a vegetable in a perfectly-OK-for-you plant oil. (If you are going to eat crisps eat the ones without the additives.)

201

3) I am showing you my fallible side – can you imagine the authors of certain world-famous, practically house-hold name, and thoroughly renowned diet books admitting they'd eaten *a potato product*? As I said at the beginning, it is almost impossible to stick to an Eating Plan for life. Which is why those on traditional diets have such a high failure rate. No point feeling guilty about it.

You will have good days and bad days. And as long as they balance out, your weight will stay the same. If you can up the number of good in proportion to the ones when you fell off the wagon you will gradually lose your excess flab.

Try to do better tomorrow.

GIVE IN TO TEMPTATION

Sometimes we really want to eat something we think is yummy. And, because we think we should lose weight, we may try to resist that thought. The problem is, the more we deny ourselves that pleasure, the more likely we are likely to be unable to think about anything else, and eventually cave in and not only eat that bun/baguette/ice-cream/pasta we've been obsessing about but all sorts of other stuff too because by then we're feeling rebellious and in sod-it mode.

So if you really want cake or chocolate or steak and kidney pudding, then have it, and balance what else you eat around it.

Sometimes I wake up and potter about and after an hour or so, this thought comes into my head: Bacon!

Once upon a time, I would have banished the notion immediately. I would have taken from the fridge a blameless but uninspiring low-fat yoghurt or some take-it-or-leave-it fruit and eaten it in a desultory and faintly hard-done-by fashion.

Now I turn the grill on. When I have a bacon feeling, I make it into a toasted sandwich with quite a lot of butter and some mustard. Sometimes I have a couple of bits of dark chocolate afterwards with my coffee (odd but true).

And recently I did that, and then had a massive piece of

coffee cake for lunch. A friend brought it round and it was just what I felt like. And did I feel guilty or concerned? I did not. Because it *is* all about balance.

The carbs were consumed early and I took them into account for the rest of the day. In the afternoon I played tennis (I lost). I had grilled halloumi, with tomatoes, basil, and a huge crunchy salad for dinner (low carb), a few peanuts with my wine, instead of crisps (protein!), and a bit more dark chocolate (it just sort of rounded things off) and then, as I do when I have any inkling that the podge might be settling in, I went for a longer walk round the block before I hit the sack.

The net result was? My weight dropped slightly. I'd had: wine, chocolate, cake, bread, bacon, and nibbles. As well as essential vitamins and minerals, some green stuff, and tomatoes.

What's not to like?

ENJOY YOURSELF

So in a vague attempt to reach a conclusion – and before my own Writer's Bottom is beyond control – I am really saying that if you want to be successful in fighting the flab, don't let it suck the pleasure from your life.

Eat foods you love, do exercise you enjoy, delight in your body – however much of it there is.

On that note, I would offer you, by way of closing comfort, some research on body shapes.

Take comfort from research.

A number of important studies – both proper university research-based and anecdotal, as well as a straw poll round my male mates – have shown that men like voluptuous females. Researchers at the University of Los Angeles (rather wasting time and money, I feel, when they could just have asked me) confirmed that while women like slim men (each to his own – personally I'd rather have a muscle-bound hunk), men like curves.

So good news for all you generously-built females and sorry chaps, but don't be too disheartened. It was LA after all.

In the real world, women, as I'm sure you know, don't much care what men look like as long as they a) make us laugh, and b) are tolerant about shopping for shoes. Big cuddly men are just fine – as long as you don't take up the entire bed and are still fit enough to carry the wine in.

The truth is, the most gorgeous, interesting, sexy people are those who are happy in their skins. And what's more likely to bring that about? Walking around light-headed from starvation, squashed into a bone-crushing corset looking at endless days of carrot juice and protein shakes?

Or having another chocolate?

(Please refer to tip one.)

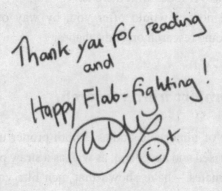

Thank you for reading and Happy Flab-fighting!

The End.
Except it isn't, quite. We're going to make it 101 …

A FAB POEM

The undisputed winner of the Fight the Flab competition, and the lucky recipient of a glorious week at Chez-Castillon in the Dordogne – that incomparable centre of creativity where the fare is served in such abundance (I like a little irony with my contests), the wine pours forth and there is a lovely chocolatier just down the road ... offers both a cautionary tale and an ingenious solution to the problem of how to fight the flab:

Ladies and Gentleman I give you:

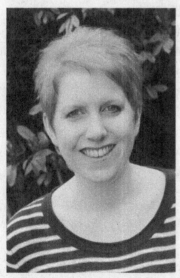

Photo by Thousand Word Media

The upside-down diet tip:
a poem by Clare Mackintosh

I was trim, I was slim,
I attended a gym,
Then I left work to become a writer.
Now I scoff, and I trough
(and I'm still no Chekhov)
It's no shock that I'm getting no lighter.
I'm game for a change, I can't stay the same,
And I've hit on the perfect idea,
It'll win, I'll be thin, I'll have only one chin,
A skinnier version of Shakespeare.
So what is the plot? It won't take a lot,
I shall stand on my head when I'm eating.
When I chew on my stew, without further ado
It'll stay in my head (that's the cheating).
Begone, deli jelly! Don't enter my belly,
Go right up and hand-feed my brain.
All that bread can instead go direct to my head,
With an order of chicken chow mein.
I shall shrink, I shall slink, I'll be able to think,
With such nutrients feeding my mind.
I shall write, I shall fight, I will not turn upright,
In my quest for a tiny behind.
The End.
P.S. Don't try this at home.

www.claremackintosh.com

RECIPES

Here are the recipes for the various delights I have mentioned throughout the book – with a couple of extras you may like to try ...

Protein-based/Eggs

Cheese soufflé

As I said, this is really easy to make – and looks great, as long as you don't open the oven door too soon and you are ready as soon as it is! If you want to impress others with your culinary skills you do need to serve it straightaway before it starts to collapse.

You can make four little ones or one larger one, but do butter the soufflé dish or ramekins thoroughly (you are doing low carb/protein/eating eggs – butter is fine!)

What you will need:
50g butter (plus whatever you need for the greasing)
50g plain flour
300ml whole milk
75g strong cheddar or grated parmesan or a mixture of both

(I like it heavy on the cheese so probably put in more than this. I am not a great measurer!)

Half teaspoon of English or a teaspoon of Dijon mustard (or a pinch of cayenne pepper)

3 large eggs, separated, plus an extra white.

What you do with it:

Heat the oven to 200°C (gas mark 6).

Do the greasing bit. (NB if you are making one big one, it is best to make a greaseproof paper collar to go round the soufflé dish to keep it in shape – grease the inside of the section that will be protruding above the dish). (NB 2 so it is probably easier to make small ones.)

Melt the butter in a saucepan and stir in the flour as if making a roux.

You will know it should be the consistency of wet sand before you add the milk, which you do gradually over a very low heat, mixing all the time with a wooden spoon until a "sauce" ensues. When thickened, remove from the heat and stir in the cheese, mustard, or cayenne, and black pepper (I throw in salt too because I put salt in everything but normal people may think the cheese makes it salty enough). If you have them, finely chopped chives are good too.

In a separate bowl, whisk up the four egg whites, as if you were making a meringue, until it goes into peaks.

Beat the egg yolks into the cheese sauce mixture and then gradually stir in the stiffened egg whites until all is combined. Divide the final mix between the ramekins, put on a baking tray, and cook in the oven for up to twenty minutes until risen and golden. Do not over-cook. Watch through the glass door if you have one, if not gently pull oven door open about an inch after 15 minutes, and peer in with one eye.

Yell at other diners that they need to get themselves in position. *Now!* For a delicious, filling, low-carb lunch or supper, serve with a Tra-La and a lovely green salad and/or a dish of thinly sliced tomatoes and onions.

(Or, if you are not in low-carb mood and would rather just skip the next meal, it's really great with some proper French bread as well.)

Chocolate mousse

While we're on eggs and protein and low carb, this makes a wonderful pudding, which has that luxurious, home-made taste but is again really simple to make. And it's quite rich so you don't need to eat much to feel as if you've had something lovely and a real treat.

What you will need:
75 –100g good, very dark, chocolate
3 large eggs
Tablespoon of rum, brandy or sherry (optional. Let it never be said that I am forcing you into bad ways).

What you do with it:
Break up the chocolate in squares and melt it over a saucepan of boiling water. (Or cheat like I do and put it in the microwave.)

While it is softening, separate the eggs.

Beat up the whites – again as if you were making a meringue – until they are stiff and stand up in peaks. Then remove the chocolate from any heat source and fold in the egg yolks, one at a time with a wooden spoon – do this gently and not if the chocolate is *too* hot – we don't want anything scrambled. When the chocolate mixture is smooth and shiny, fold the whites into this. Again, be gentle. When thoroughly combined and a uniform colour, pour into serving dishes – you can use ramekins again (if they're not full of cheese soufflé) or the mousse looks pretty in round wine glasses.

Chill down in the fridge. Decorate with whipped cream if desired, and some grated chocolate if you want it to look nice.

NB you can make a creamier, milder version (which kids might prefer) by adding whipped cream to the mixture at the same time as the egg whites.

Yum.

Going Raw

Jane's raw veg mountain

What you will need:
A mountain of raw veg. What you choose to include is infinitely variable – walk into your local greengrocer's or up the fruit and veg aisle in the supermarket (Waitrose is particularly good if you want a fine selection of exotic vegetation) and see what grabs your eye. Basically if you can eat it raw, go for it.
I like to use all or some of these:
Red, green, and yellow peppers (diced)
A finely chopped chilli (of course!)

A bunch of asparagus (woody ends removed, chopped into small cylinders)

Spring onions – (remove end bits and hairy tops then ditto)

White or red cabbage (shredded)

Carrots (grated)

Any number of green leaves, including fresh coriander and basil

An avocado, taken out of its skin and diced.

You might also like to chop up: radishes, celery, sugar snap peas, cucumber, or green beans

Some diet gurus advise against eating cabbage (and also spinach) raw as they claim it can block the production of thyroid hormones. Others are all for it, claiming that raw cruciferous veg (cabbage, broccoli, kale, sprouts etc) can actually protect against some cancers. I wouldn't know. All I can say is that I'm pretty sure the odd cup of coleslaw won't do you much harm …

What you do with it:

Trim, chop, grate, shred as necessary, pile on plate (excess veg can be stored in airtight containers or plastic bags in the fridge till next time).

I use a simple dressing made from extra virgin olive oil, balsamic vinegar, a pinch of mustard powder, dried oregano, and salt and black pepper, all well shaken-up. (You can add crushed garlic – also v good for you – to this, if you like garlic and don't have to breathe over anyone.)

I drizzle the dressing all over the veg, then add some dollops of houmous, roughly mix, and munch. You will be amazed at how filling it can be.

213

NB the addition of the shop-bought houmous is cheating slightly, as the chick peas have been cooked, but the rest is all raw, so what the hell. Houmous makes it taste really nice …

Sunflower pâté (kindly supplied by Alison Matthews of Raw Confidence)

(I tried this and it is fine but I'm not huge on sundried tomatoes, if you are, you'll like it)

What you will need:

Cup of sunflower seeds

¼ cup sundried tomatoes

¼ teaspoon of paprika

Salt if required

Water as required

What you do with it:

Blend all the ingredients together to form a pâté, adding the water gradually so it doesn't become too runny.

Serve with crudités, oatcakes, rice cakes, or salad. Can also be stuffed into small peppers or put on top of raw mushrooms. Will keep in the fridge for a few days.

Walnut pâté (as above)

(I did not try this because I cannot abide walnuts, but if you love 'em – why not … good protein snack as well as being raw!)

What you will need:

1 cup walnuts soaked overnight

2 tablespoons olive oil

½ teaspoon of mixed spice (add more if required)

1 clove garlic

Salt if required

Water as required

What you do with it:

Blend all the ingredients together to make a paste, again being careful with the water so the mixture doesn't become too runny.

Will keep in the fridge for a few days.

Raw chocolate truffles – also suggested by Alison Matthews.

(I have had these – generously made for me by my Go-raw volunteer guinea pig, Paula. I loved them.)

What you will need:

50g raw cacao butter

100g raw cacao powder

100g finely ground almonds

1 teaspoon vanilla essence or 1 vanilla pod

Agave or honey to taste (probably around 1-2 tablespoons)

Small pinch of salt (to taste)

What you do with it:

Shave the cacao butter into slivers and melt in a bowl over a saucepan of hot water (not boiling). Heat very slowly or the temperature will be too high and your truffles will no longer be raw, even though they will still taste great!

Take the melted cacao butter off the heat and mix in the cacao powder and ground almonds. You can do this in a blender if you prefer. Add the vanilla and some of the agave or honey and salt and taste. Add more sweetener if you wish.

Roll into small balls and put in the fridge for 30 minutes to set.

Will keep in the fridge for about half an hour! ☺

Being healthy

Janie's fantastic salads

I've made much of the wonderful food at Chez-Castillon, where I teach in the Dordogne. Here's an example of the sort of dishes that taste so thoroughly delightful and moreish but that are still made up of really healthy stuff.

Salads are a particular forte of the Chez-Castillon kitchen and Janie Millman, chief cook and bottle-washer, has a real knack for putting together colours and flavours. Last time I was there I particularly loved her simple salad of diced beetroot, feta cheese, almonds, white wine vinegar, olive oil, lemon juice, and cumin – a combination of ingredients that worked beautifully, and I begged for the details of how to make this:

A great spicy chicken salad
What you will need:

Chicken breast

Mayonnaise

Chopped chillies

Flakes of parmesan

Onions

Fresh coriander leaves

Pine nuts or crushed
cashews

Lardons

Rocket leaves

Fresh tomatoes

Olive oil

Lemon juice

White wine vinegar

Dijon mustard

What you do with it:

Janie first dices up the chicken breast into quite small pieces
and fries them in a little olive oil with the chopped chilli,
onion, and pine nuts together with some lardons.

She then mixes together the rocket or spinach, with some
chopped fresh tomatoes and crushed nuts and dresses it with
a blend of olive oil, white wine vinegar, a teaspoon of Dijon
mustard, a table spoonful of mayonnaise, and the juice of
half a lemon.

The hot chicken is then spooned straight onto the rocket
leaves so they wilt a little, and Janie then tops the whole
dish off with flakes of parmesan cheese and fresh coriander
leaves …

It is delicious!

And, as Janie says, as a recipe it is also endlessly adaptable. Substitute the rocket for uncooked spinach, use tinned chickpeas in place of, or as well as, the nuts and try hot peppery chorizo if you prefer, instead of lardons.

The point is that you end up with a generous helping of stuff that tastes fantastic, is really good for you, and – I promise you – is filling and will leave you suitably replete.

Remember what we said earlier about not shoving it down at speed. Relax, munch, enjoy. Sip some white wine with it. Bask in that virtuous glow …

Janie makes a mean pasta sauce too. But she said if I passed that on, she'd have to kill me, so that one is still up my sleeve …

Instead, and much less excitingly, we will move on to:

Soups for all seasons

The basic cabbage soup recipe

(I'm not sure how long this is supposed to last you but it makes quite a lot …)

What you will need:
6 large onions 2 green peppers 2 tins of tomatoes (chopped or whole)
250g fresh mushrooms 1 bunch celery
½ head cabbage
3 carrots 1 packet dry onion soup mix
1 or 2 stock cubes
Salt and pepper

Cayenne pepper, curry powder, chilli, or mixed herbs to your taste.

What you do with it:
Use spray oil to sauté the chopped onions in a large pot.
Add the green pepper pieces and heat for a minute.
Add the chopped cabbage leaves, sliced carrots, celery, and mushrooms.
Sprinkle over a little cayenne pepper or curry powder.
Add 12 cups of water and any additional stock cubes.
Cook over a medium heat until the vegetables are tender and the soup is the right consistency.
(I am not imbued with excitement – are you?)

Quick no-fat soup (aka Katie's red soup)
This is based on something that Katie Fforde makes, which she calls her "red soup", which is quick to make and good to fill yourself up with without taking in many calories.

What you will need:
A packet of mixed frozen veg (e.g. the sort that contains a selection of peas, beans, swede, carrot, sweetcorn, broccoli florets, cauliflower, etc.)
A tin of tomatoes (chopped may be easier but whole can soon be mashed up)
Stock or stock cubes (Katie likes the jelly ones)
Water (I'm also adding a splash of wine)
Chilli, herbs, spices, seasonings, according to taste.

What you do with it:

Tip the vegetables into a large saucepan with the tin of tomatoes, some water, stock, and seasoning and simmer until the vegetables are tender. You can then either eat it "lumpy" as Katie does, or whiz it up in the blender until it's smooth. I quite like soups to be a combination of both sometimes – you can always whiz up half of it, but keep half the lumps back for texture.

That's the really low calorie version.

Variations are to add a little pasta or rice or a couple of potatoes, to bulk it out and make it more filling. I like soup with grated cheese sprinkled on top too. As Katie says, this "tastes nice, is filling, and feels quite wicked as it involves pasta/rice/cheese." She also adds a lot of chilli.

Quite right too.

For a more luxurious and slightly more calorific version, start by sweating onions and garlic in a little olive oil and butter, then add a selection of chopped vegetables, including potato, and a definite splash of wine, cook till soft, whiz up, swirl in a little cream or fromage frais and a drop of sherry. Serve with grated cheese for sure, a sprinkling of fresh herbs, lots of black pepper (and chopped chillies for me).

But even with this one, you can knock it back all day and get away with it.

My fish soup

I don't know whether you like fish soup but I fell in love with it after spending time in Normandy and spent some considerable time back home trying to recreate the fragrant broth I had had there. With grated cheese, garlicky croutons, and a generous dollop of aioli it makes a whole meal. This is how I make mine:

What you will need:

A selection of fishbones, heads, tails and any leftover fish (if you've had grilled fish on the bone for dinner for example, keep everybody's remains! Otherwise your local fishmonger or fish counter will oblige if you ask them nicely.)

Some fish flesh (although strangely this is not essential!)

1 large potato (diced – I don't bother to peel)

2 onions (peeled and chopped)

1 clove garlic (crushed)

I tin chopped tomatoes

1 tbsp tomato puree

Mixed dried herbs

Fresh parsley

Salt and black pepper

Dry white wine

Olive oil and butter

What you do with it:

Heat a splosh (a tablespoon or two) of the olive oil and a generous knob of butter in a large, heavy saucepan over a low heat and when the butter has foamed, add half the onions and garlic. Cook gently till the onions soften and melt. Add all

221

the fishy bits (less any fillets of flesh you are using) and continue to fry. Add in any other stray bits of veg you've got hanging around that you want to get rid of – carrots etc – keep stirring and when it's all threatening to stick, deglaze with a large glass of wine and have couple of mouthfuls yourself (one of the joys of cooking with wine is that you get to check it hasn't gone off). Top up with cold water until all the ingredients are covered, add salt and pepper and the tomato puree (it makes it look prettier when you're staring at fish eyes) and leave to simmer for at least an hour but the longer the better (all day is good if the aroma of fish market won't upset you) and the more intense the flavour. (I have left bones in a slow-cooker all night before now).

Eventually when it has all boiled down to a mush and the bones have fallen apart, remove from the heat, strain, and discard all solids. (If you live by the sea – and you put this on a flowerbed in the garden, the seagulls will make short work of it! Saves making the bin smell.)

Reserve the fish stock, reheat your heavy saucepan with some more butter and oil and soften the rest of the onions and garlic. Add the diced potato and cook slowly for ten minutes till the potatoes have begun to soften. Add tomatoes, salt and pepper, and herbs – fresh basil leaves can be nice too if you have them. Pour in the fish stock and simmer until the potato is completely cooked.

If you are using some skinned fillets of fish (and if you've made your stock strong enough, you don't need to) you've now got two options. You can cut them up into small pieces and drop them in now, cook for a minute or two until they are done – fish cooks in no time – and then whiz up (those hand-held blenders are brilliant) the whole lot for a totally smooth soup, with a fishy body. Or you can do the blending first and then poach the small pieces of soup in the liquid and leave them to be eaten whole. You can drop a few frozen prawns in at the same time for an extra hearty dish.

Either way, check the seasoning and add salt and a good grind of black pepper as necessary. Finish off with swirl of cream, a dash of sherry, fresh parsley if wanted, and serve with loads of crisp croutons (make your own by brushing cubes of bread with olive oil and crisping in a very hot oven or frying pan or do the low-fat version of basically cutting up very well done toast) and lashings of grated cheese. If it's a feed-your-face-day have aioli as well. Sounds a palava but honestly if you get it right, it tastes bloody marvellous!

Total indulgence

And talking of marvellous …

The perfect egg-mayo sandwich
The unrivalled joy of eating a really good sandwich is the reason I could never give up bread for ever. I think eggs make the best one of all though a tuna or chicken mayonnaise can be pretty good too, if made with love.

What you will need:
Good bread (none of your white, additive-ridden pap. Make it yourself, get it from a proper baker's, or buy from the high end of the supermarket offerings. I like Granary best)

Butter (the real thing)

Eggs (free-range, of course!)

Mayonnaise, salt and pepper.

I'm never sure how much cress brings to the party – though I'm happy to eat it – but shredded basil leaves are rather good. (You can also use raw spinach.)

What you do with it:

Boil your eggs (if this isn't teaching you to suck them) – but not for too long. Slightly sloppy makes for a better sandwich than all overdone and granular.

Mash them up with lots of mayonnaise, and salt and black pepper. Add the shredded basil leaves to the bowl now so they are evenly distributed and give them a good mix in to spread the flavour. (Sometimes I put a finely-chopped chilli in too but I didn't mention it in case you think I've got a fixation.)

Butter the bread, pile the egg on (do not skimp). Add the top slice – cut into *triangles* (it is true, they do taste better) and arrange beautifully on a plate with cherry tomatoes (if you like your booze you may be low on potassium) and lots of *good* (the hand-fried type) crisps! Open a chilled white wine or a bottle of fizz and sit back and enjoy.

Remember we are chewing slowly, savouring every mouthful, doing away with guilt, and allowing ourselves to eat things we like.

Which is why as long as you promise to walk before bed, you can also have a chocolate …

A proper box of chocolates:
What you will need:
Your favourite selection. I'm quite partial to Terry's All Gold, almost anything by Hotel Chocolat or a good Belgian selection in plain[9] …

What you do with it:
Eat them one at a time. Set yourself a challenge to see how long you can make them last. You're having chocolates, right? You don't need to eat the whole layer. (If you do – starve tomorrow).

Proper roast potatoes
I mentioned goose fat and this does undoubtedly make the best roast potatoes. I was going to hold forth on the secret behind the perfect golden, crusty, goose-fat roasted spud but I have decided to keep my powder dry in readiness for the *Fight-the-Flab Complete Recipe Collection* for which, no doubt, there will soon be feverish clamourings from my eager readership.

Until then, thanks for reading this one.

And Happy Flab-fighting!

Footnote 9 my birthday is in January.

Notes

Notes

Notes

Notes

Notes

Notes

OTHER BOOKS
YOU COULD READ:

The 5:2 Diet Book by Kate Harrison (Orion) *How to lose weight via intermittent fasting*

The Fast Diet by Michael Moseley (Short Books) *The science behind intermittent fasting explained and in action*

Burn Fat Fast: The alternate-day low-GL diet plan by Patrick Holford (Piatkus) *Another angle on intermittent fasting*

The Carbohydrate Addict's Diet Book by Dr Rachel F. Heller and Dr Richard F Heller (Vermilion) *Worth a try if you can't curb the carbs*

Food for Heroes – the official Help for Heroes Cook Book (Accent Press) *Celebrity recipes in a good cause*

The Manorama Formula by M. Legha (Grafton) (currently out of print but available second-hand) *Fascinating theories about self-regulation and weight-control*

The MILF Diet by Jessica Porter (Atria Books) *"Gain a spicier sex life and find your inner goddess" – with whole grains*

Fat Chance: The Bitter Truth about Sugar by Robert Lustig (Fourth Estate) *Why it's worth cutting down on the sweet stuff*

The Sweet Poison Quit Plan by David Gillespie (Penguin) *How to do just that*

The Sober Revolution by Sarah Turner and Lucy Rocca (Accent Press) *If it's time to cut back on the wine*
Raising the Roof a novel by Jane Wenham-Jones (that's me!) (Transworld) *The Story of The Shelf Diet*
Any other book by Jane Wenham-Jones – *every little helps*

Websites: www.100waystofighttheflab.com
http://janewenhamjones.wordpress.com

Acknowledgements:

My heartfelt thanks for help, tips, contributions, and support go to: Stephen Arkell, Morgen Bailey, Janice Biggs, Michaella Bolder, Karen Booth, Felicity Brookesmith, Chez-Castillon Creative Writing Courses, Teresa Chris, The Cocoa Exchange, Sarah Duncan, Paula Erol, Zacchary Falconer-Barfield, Katie Fforde, Lynne Hackles, Judith Haire, Bill Harris, Kate Harrison, David Headley, Cathy Lennon, Jane Lovering, Clare Mackintosh, Alison Matthews, Carol Midgley, Janie Millman, Betty Orme, Tony Tibbenham, Shirley Webb and Tom Wenham-Jones.

With special appreciation for Cat Camacho, Stephanie Williams, Hazel Cushion, Alison Stokes and all at Accent Press.

Chocolate all round . . .